P9-DHL-174

Acknowledgments

The following wonderful people—some health-care professionals and some parents of "sweet kids"—reviewed the first edition of our book. Without them, we couldn't have produced the book you're holding. Thanks to Nathaniel Clark, MD, RD, CDE, for reviewing the second edition.

JoAnn Ahern, RN, MSN, CS, CDE
New Haven, Connecticut

Jean Betschart Roemer, MN, RN, CDE
Pittsburgh, Pennsylvania

Keith Campbell, RPh, MBA, CDE
Pullman, Washington

Tess Curran
Phoenix, Arizona

Kim Heintzman, MS, RD, LD, CDE
Albuquerque, New Mexico

Ann Hussey
Wantagh, New York

Donna Jornsay, RN, CDE
Great Neck, New York

Gloria Loring
Los Angeles, California

Joyce Mosiman, RD, LD, CDE
Kansas City, Missouri

Joyce Green Pastors, RD, MS, CDE
Charlottesville, Virginia

Leslie Plotnick, MD
Baltimore, Maryland

Stephanie Schwartz, RN, MPH, CDE
Kansas City, Missouri

Susan Thom, RN, LD, CDE
Brecksville, Ohio

sweet kids

SECOND EDITION

Betty Page Brackenridge, MS, RD, CDE

Richard R. Rubin, PhD, CDE

▲®American Diabetes Association®

Cure • Care • Commitment℠

Director, Book Publishing, John Fedor; *Associate Director, Consumer Books,* Sherrye Landrum; *Editor,* Mary Beth Oelkers-Keegan; *Production Manager,* Peggy M. Rote; *Composition,* Circle Graphics, Inc.; *Cover Design,* Design Literate, Inc.; *Printer,* Transcontinental Printing Inc.

Printed in Canada
1 3 5 7 9 10 8 6 4 2

The suggestions and information contained in this publication are generally consistent with the *Clinical Practice Recommendations* and other policies of the American Diabetes Association, but they do not represent the policy or position of the Association or any of its boards or committees. Reasonable steps have been taken to ensure the accuracy of the information presented. However, the American Diabetes Association cannot ensure the safety or efficacy of any product or service described in this publication. Individuals are advised to consult a physician or other appropriate health care professional before undertaking any diet or exercise program or taking any medication referred to in this publication. Professionals must use and apply their own professional judgment, experience, and training and should not rely solely on the information contained in this publication before prescribing any diet, exercise, or medication. The American Diabetes Association—its officers, directors, employees, volunteers, and members—assumes no responsibility or liability for personal or other injury, loss, or damage that may result from the suggestions or information in this publication.

⊗ The paper in this publication meets the requirements of the ANSI Standard Z39.48-1992 (permanence of paper).

ADA titles may be purchased for business or promotional use or for special sales. For information, please write to Lee Romano Sequeira, Special Sales & Promotions, at the address below.

American Diabetes Association
1701 North Beauregard Street
Alexandria, Virginia 22311

Library of Congress Cataloging-in-Publication Data

Brackenridge, Betty Page, 1946-
    Sweet kids: how to balance diabetes control and good nutrition with family peace /
Betty Page Brackenridge and Richard R. Rubin.—[2nd ed.]
      p.   cm.
    Includes index.
    ISBN 1-58040-124-4 (pbk. : alk. paper)
    Diabetes in children—Diet therapy. 2. Children—Nutrition. I. Rubin, Richard R.
  II. Title.
RJ420.D5 B726 2002
    618.92'4620654—dc21   2002019585

Contents

What Diabetes Can Do to Families

I'd been in my first job as a dietitian for only a few weeks when I got my first lesson in what diabetes can do to families. It came from Josh Taylor and his mother, Nancy. Josh was a handsome little eight-year-old with bright red hair and freckles. With his jeans, oversized striped T-shirt, and sneakers, he looked like the all-American boy. Mom, on the other hand, looked like a poster child for parental stress. She seemed worried and exhausted. She had deep circles under her big blue eyes, and her mouth was a thin, tight line.

Josh's family had just joined the health plan where I worked. Because Josh's growth had slowed down, the pediatrician sent him to see me so I could "adjust the calorie level" of his diabetes meal plan. The idea was to provide enough calories to get his growth back on track. But it soon became clear that there was much more going on than simply an outgrown meal plan: Josh and his family were battling over food up to six times a day. And the struggles had been getting worse.

Diabetes arrives on the scene like a gorilla at the symphony— impossible to ignore!

According to his mother, the amount of food on the meal plan was never quite right. Sometimes Josh wasn't very hungry. When that happened, she made him stay at the table until he cleaned his plate. She hated to do it because it made him so unhappy, but she just couldn't think of any other way to get him to eat. Sometimes he would still be sitting at the dinner table when bedtime arrived.

When Josh's blood sugar was really low before supper and she knew he had to eat something, she confessed that she would bribe him to finish a meal—offering him extra allowance money, toys, and even movie tickets for cleaning his plate.

Josh said he thought it was worse when he was still hungry after a meal. Sometimes he begged for more food, but his parents almost always refused. They believed they had to follow the meal plan to the letter for Josh's own good. They told him he could have "free" foods, like calorie-free gelatin or raw vegetables, since those wouldn't raise his blood sugar. But he usually refused these and sulked until snack time.

They both agreed that the biggest battle happened when Mom found a stash of candy bars and snack cakes in the back of Josh's closet. To hear them talk about it, the explosion must have been impressive.

I was flabbergasted by their troubles. My training just hadn't prepared me for what Josh and his family were going through. They hadn't enjoyed a peaceful meal in months. Josh resisted every effort to control his eating. Even worse, he was angry with his father and brother for eating the sweets he was now being denied.

These were nice, intelligent people doing their best to follow orders. The meal plan that their previous doctor and dietitian had given them specified food choices, portion sizes, and the timing of meals, but the struggle to follow the plan exactly was taking a heavy toll on them. And to make matters worse, all that effort and heartache hadn't even kept Josh's blood sugar under control. He was having low blood sugars several times a week, his hemoglobin A1C was 11.6 percent, and he had nearly stopped growing.

In the years since I first met Josh's family, I have learned a lot about the problems that can follow diabetes into the family circle. Shots may be frightening at first. Blood tests can be uncomfortable and expensive. Worries about complications are always somewhere in the background. But as hard as these things are, I believe that food is often the most difficult thing for families to deal with. This is partly because food can be an issue at almost any moment (not just a few times a day, like shots and tests). In addition, food has personal, cultural, and social meaning. That's why food issues are often highly emotional. As diabetes intrudes into this important area, arguments about food can disrupt the daily life and harmony of the family.

After all, food is the very stuff of life. Eating the right type and amount of food is essential to growth, from birth to maturity. The feelings and activities that surround eating give children their first lessons about life. Food is such an important part of a child's life that mealtime experiences can color her whole world. Food is intimately involved in physical, mental, and emotional development and, ultimately, in the child's successful growth into a separate, independent adult.

If a hungry infant is fed in a close and relaxed way, she learns that the world is a safe place. When feeding progresses normally, the child then learns to trust herself as she begins to choose her own foods and to notice and respond to her body's signals of hunger and satisfaction. Decision-making skills, self-confidence, and positive self-image should all develop naturally at the family table.

When parents can relax and just do their job, eating is handled in a matter-of-fact fashion. Mom and Dad put suitable foods on the table and model how people are expected to eat and behave in their particular family. In a friendly, low-key atmosphere, taste and appetite help each member decide what and how much to eat. Foods are chosen not only for their nutritional value but also because they add to the family's enjoyment and are an expression of its culture. In a family that isn't obsessed with food, kids who aren't particularly hungry on one night eat less than usual. If they're terribly hungry another night, they eat more. No big deal.

But when diabetes arrives on the scene, like a gorilla at the symphony, it's impossible to ignore! Imagine what would happen if a great ape walked into a concert hall. As one musician and then another notices the gorilla, everything starts to fall apart. Music stands get knocked over. Nobody watches the conductor. The gorilla throws banana peels on the stage and grabs the wigs off the startled heads of well-dressed ladies. No more concert. Just a confused jumble of noise. People leave the concert hall with their minds in an uproar and the scent of bananas clinging to their clothes.

A silly picture, I admit. But it's also a pretty good image of how diabetes can confuse the very basic process of getting a family fed, nurtured, and civilized. Parents do difficult and sometimes painful things because of their own worries and their healthcare providers' expectations. They often try to control with a clock and a measuring cup what is meant to unfold naturally from a child's appetite and pattern of growth and development. The normal progression of a child choosing his own food as he grows older may be drastically slowed or even stopped. Mom and Dad become the "food police." Power struggles follow. Families go to war over how many vanilla wafers were eaten after school. The effect on relationships, development, and stress levels can be overwhelming.

But it is possible to ease these worries and regain sanity. Pleasant meals are not out of reach.

Richard Rubin and I originally wrote this book to help families dealing with diabetes develop confidence and a measure of humor, especially around the central issue of food. Some years have passed since we wrote the first edition, and many changes have occurred in the diabetes world. The equipment used to monitor blood sugars has improved, so it's not as uncomfortable and as much of a hassle to use. Rapid-acting insulin has come into wide use, dramatically changing the business of balancing food and insulin. In addition, when we wrote the first edition, the use of insulin pumps was limited almost entirely to adults. Now more kids than ever are using pumps; in fact, their use is growing more rapidly among kids than in any other group. This new edition covers these and other changes in the diabetes landscape.

But much about diabetes hasn't changed, so all the practical information about families, behavior, and nutrition from the first edition is still here. The resulting blend of old and new is meant to help real families in the real world.

Throughout *Sweet Kids,* you'll find stories about families like yours. Some of them are funny, others sad. But all are stories of the strength, creativity, wisdom, and love of families trying to live the best life possible while dealing with the realities of diabetes. It has been a privilege working with these families over the years, and it has also been the best schooling in the world. And everything we've learned, you'll find in this book.

It would be easy to gawk at the gorilla and forget the symphony. It's also easy to become so focused on diabetes that your child's other needs, as well as your own, never get proper attention. If the joy of eating and preparing food has disappeared, spontaneity seems lost forever, or you're just looking for some new ideas on how to cope with food and diabetes, please read on.

RICHARD R. RUBIN

When It's Your Child with Diabetes

April 2, 1979. I sat with my seven-year-old son, Stefan, as his pediatrician confirmed what I had suspected for the past few weeks: Stefan had diabetes. The signs had all been there. The constant thirst and urination, the tremendous hunger, and finally, the home urine glucose test that read 4+. (Back then, urine sugar testing was all we had. Blood sugar testing didn't arrive until a couple of years later.)

As we sat there listening to Dr. Bill tell us all the ways in which our lives were about to change, I felt nervous, even downright scared. My thoughts turned to a day almost exactly 20 years earlier, when my sister Mary Sue, then nine years old, was diagnosed with diabetes. Her diabetes had been hard for my family. We didn't talk about it much. But in a way, that only made matters worse. I could see her stress as she tested, gave herself shots with those old glass syringes that had to be boiled before each use, sharpened the needles so her shots wouldn't hurt so much, and made the

I felt overwhelmed, and I desperately wanted not to feel that way.

myriad daily adjustments that had become a part of her life now that she had diabetes.

I could also remember the pressure diabetes placed on my parents. They worked hard to make sure that Mary Sue ate exactly the right amount of exactly the right foods at exactly the right time. They did a good job, but it also meant that life was very tightly structured at our house.

Those memories darted through my mind on that early April morning in the doctor's office. I felt overwhelmed, and I desperately wanted not to feel that way. I wanted to feel strong. I wanted to feel confident that Stefan and I and the whole family could take diabetes in stride, that we could cope, that our lives could remain wonderful. But I had my doubts. I needed some sign that we would be okay. And then Dr. Bill turned to me and said, "Okay, Dick, now you pull down your pants. I want you to stick yourself with this syringe to show Stefan that it doesn't hurt too much." Suddenly, this crazy thought went through my mind: "Well, at least I'm wearing clean underwear!"

Then I laughed for the first time in weeks. I told Bill and Stefan what I'd been thinking, and they laughed, too. The tension eased a little for all of us, and my confidence that we could cope was restored. Naturally, this was only the first step on the never-ending road that all families living with diabetes must travel. It was a crucial step, nonetheless. I believed we could manage, even before I knew exactly how we would do it.

From the moment Stefan's diabetes was diagnosed, I tried to learn as much as I could about this disease and its management. I talked to Stefan's healthcare team and lots of other diabetes providers. I read books. We attended classes. Everything I read and learned kept coming back to the same point: "If your child eats right, exercises, and takes his insulin, he (and you) can lead a perfectly normal life." Much as I wanted to believe this, experience quickly taught me it simply wasn't true. That's not to say our life was bleak, because it wasn't. It was still full and exciting. In many ways, it was even more exciting than it had been before diabetes. But normal it wasn't.

How can life with diabetes be normal when you are constantly planning and adjusting, worrying and readjusting? Many parents say that the early stages of life with diabetes remind them of what it was like to have a new baby. Among other things, you've always got to carry stuff to deal with potential emergencies. Only now, instead of toting bottles and diapers and baby wipes, it's snacks and syringes, insulin and blood sugar meters.

Many of the adjustments you make when your child gets diabetes are related to food. That's not surprising, since food and eating touch every waking moment. Food is different from other aspects of diabetes care. Once your child has taken his shot or tested his blood sugar, no one needs to worry about those things until the next time. The same is true of exercise. But at any moment of the day, your child can eat too much or too little, or eat the wrong things. Moreover, you have to somehow coordinate your child's food needs with those of the rest of your family.

In the first months after Stefan's diabetes was diagnosed, we worked hard to get his eating just right, just as my parents had done with my sister 20 years earlier. We weighed and measured and struggled to memorize the American Diabetes Association's dietary exchange lists. Looking back, I see that all of this was helpful. It gave us a solid foundation on which to build our own unique structure for life with diabetes—a structure that suited our lifestyle and our son's need to grow up as healthy and normal as possible.

Since 1979, I've worked with many families who are living with diabetes, and I've learned from all of them. They have taught me how powerfully a child's diabetes can affect family life. I've also learned how creatively and beautifully some families manage the challenge. And, perhaps most important of all, I've learned *how* they do it. The guidelines and suggestions offered in this book are drawn from that experience. In *Sweet Kids,* Betty Brackenridge and I share with you all the practical lessons we have learned over the years.

My greatest teacher is still my son Stefan. He is living proof that it is possible to grow up healthy and strong with diabetes. Today Stefan is a young man, and a father himself. May your child flourish as wonderfully as he has!

1

What Parents Can Do to Promote Healthy Eating

Picture 15-month-old Lucy and her mother in their cheerful yellow kitchen. Ginger, the baby's mother, has spread a big blue shower curtain under the highchair and covered the stove top and canister set with plaid dishtowels. She's wearing her husband's barbecue apron over her clothes. Lucy is stripped down to the bare essentials: diaper and bib. It's time for lunch, and it isn't going to be pretty.

The older the baby got, the more creative she became at avoiding unwanted food.

When Lucy developed diabetes at eight months of age, she was happily eating rice cereal and milled carrots and was still breast-feeding. As Ginger described those times, her face lit up with a grin. Nursing had created islands of calm in their busy days. She and Lucy cheerfully snuggled through most feedings, unaware of their surroundings. As for solid foods, Ginger said, "Sometimes Lucy didn't eat a whole lot, but she always smiled and chattered at me. I could tell when she'd had enough. She'd clamp the spoon between her gums and give me a wicked little smile." That was before diabetes.

The first big change had been to do away with breast-feeding. The dietitian said there was no way to tell if Lucy was getting enough. Formula would be "much easier to keep track of." Reluctantly, Ginger agreed. The transition hadn't been easy. It was one more change to deal with at an already difficult time. Insulin shots, blood glucose testing, worry, grief. It had all been so hard. "Someday I'll write a book," she told me.

Each feeding was planned to provide a certain number of ounces of formula and one or two servings of cereal, fruit, vegetables, or meat. Ginger dutifully began trying to make Lucy eat it all. But the more she forced, the less Lucy ate. Their struggle escalated as Mom got more and more desperate. The baby responded by going on the offensive. The fur (and the food) began to fly. Until Ginger thought of using that shower curtain, she had been washing the floor, walls, and counters after every meal.

Lucy still clamped her jaw down when she'd had enough. But now, Ginger would try various tricks to get those last few bites down her throat. Mom would begin with the make-believe choo-choo train or airplane deliveries of baby food. Eventually, she'd sink to prying the child's mouth open and shoveling the food in. The older the baby got, the more creative she became at avoiding unwanted food. Spitting, spilling, throwing, smearing: She became a true artist at keeping the offending items from reaching her stomach. Mom swore that Lucy stayed cheerful about the whole situation. But she herself wasn't in the same frame of mind.

"I'm not sure that it's worth the struggle," Ginger said. "Her blood sugars are a mess anyway. I'm tempted to just forget the whole thing: to let Lucy eat what she wants and then try to keep up with it as best I can."

Ginger was frustrated and exhausted. Even so, she and Lucy were doing much better than a lot of families. What made the difference was the fact that Lucy was keeping her cool. That's not usually the case in situations like this.

Typically, when children are forced to eat, they become angry and fight back. They may cry, scream, and squirm. And the ugly emotional response often makes parents force even harder. The war escalates. "Eat it or else!" "You can't leave the table until all those noodles are gone!" It's no fun, and it's a no-win situation for all concerned. These battles seldom produce the desired effect. When the smoke clears, everybody is irritated and exhausted—and the food is often sitting there uneaten anyway.

Do You Know Your Job Description?

Lucy's balky response to her mom's strong-arm tactics was predictable. It happened because Mom overstepped the bounds of her job description. You may not believe that there are food-related job descriptions for parents and kids, but there are. Trouble almost always results when those roles aren't played out as they should be.

Where food and eating are concerned, the roles are nicely summarized by an old cliché: "You can lead a horse to water, but you can't make him drink." Simply put, parents are supposed to provide the food. Kids then decide whether or not to eat it. We know this may sound unreasonable, and even unsafe, at first. But helping your child internalize control over food choices and amounts is an important key to lifelong health and better diabetes control.

Hunger and thirst are internal: internal to a horse at the watering trough as well as to a child at the dinner table. No one can tell from the outside whether a child is hungry or thirsty on the inside—no well-meaning parent and certainly no doctor or dietitian sitting in an office miles from home. Kids eventually get old enough to tell us what they're feeling. Unfortunately, even when they do, we sometimes ignore them.

At one time or another, nearly all parents (with or without the unique pressures of diabetes) attempt to control how much their children eat. Sometimes they try to force them to eat more and other times they try to withhold food. Their parents did it to them and they continue the tradition. Unfortunately, it usually does not work.

Forcing Children to Eat Doesn't Work

Forcing children to eat usually backfires because it violates a perfectly good internal system of control. Your reluctant gourmet may eat sooner or later, mostly because you've been fighting for so long that she eventually does get hungry. But forcing food often produces an angry or beaten child who ends up eating less than she would have if left alone. And it wears out the parents.

Cleaning your plate has been a big issue between parents and children for a long time. Some parents and grandparents are still affected by memories of the Depression or of food rationing during World War II. Still others emigrated from countries where starvation was widespread. During these and other hard times, it was important to eat everything you could when food was available. The truth was that it might not be around if you waited. And so, for as long as we can remember, children have been urged repeatedly and forcefully to "clean that plate." The specific history may be different, but the behavior is familiar throughout the world.

Many methods have been used to enforce the clean plate policy. Some of us were told how much the food had cost our hard-working parents. Others got the line, "Waste not, want not." Countless kids heard about the plight of the poor starving children in various third-world countries. And myriad moppets were simply left to sit there until late into the night—"You're not leaving this table until you eat that perfectly good liver and Brussels sprouts!"

One unintended effect of that kind of pressure is to teach kids to ignore or doubt what their own bodies are telling them. This is one reason why some adults have trouble controlling their food intake. They never learned to eat when they're hungry and stop when they're full. Instead, they tend to eat because of things outside themselves— the time of day, the presence of food, social pressure, or the desire to please others. These things effect everyone's food choices to some extent, but for some, the feelings are even stronger than their own hunger and satisfaction.

Withholding Food from Hungry Kids Doesn't Work Either

Today, some parents limit food, even when kids are still hungry. The main reason seems to be the immense value that our culture now places on being thin. As a result, parents can be tempted or, sadly, encouraged by physicians to place children on diets, withholding food that the child wants or even food needed for normal, complete nutrition. This is a more risky and complicated issue than it seems to be at first glance. If you are concerned about weight, weight loss, or body type in your children, we urge you to read *How to Get Your Kid to Eat . . . But Not Too Much* by Ellyn Satter (Bull Publishing, Palo Alto, CA, 1987) for some excellent practical advice.

Diabetes can encourage both types of controlling behavior. Parents sometimes feel compelled to make their children eat more to prevent lows. At other times, they prevent kids from eating all they want because of concerns about blood sugar or weight. Trying to manage food in these ways seems logical, but it doesn't work in the long run.

Follow the Job Description to Reach Long-Term Goals

If parents always try to control foods chosen and amounts eaten, children will have a hard time learning to do it for themselves. And if your child doesn't learn to manage her own eating now, she may never learn.

And if there's one skill that's vital to a child with diabetes, it's learning to manage food successfully. She'll need that skill all her life to feel well and stay healthy. She won't get to that point if you control choices and portions throughout childhood, or turn eating into a battle, and then say, "Now it's your job, dear," when she turns 18.

The process starts in infancy and proceeds through predictable stages until one day she is able to manage her own nutrition. Babies, toddlers, and preschoolers begin to learn food patterns and preferences as they pick and eat their fill from the foods their parents provide. School-age children choose, sometimes wisely, sometimes not, from the wider variety of foods available outside the family home. And finally, teenagers become able to plan meals for themselves and others, hopefully without dooming anyone to scurvy or a heart attack. Not that they'll do these things perfectly at any stage. But they will be capable of making their own choices and, eventually, of doing at least as good a job as the rest of us.

Trying to control your child's diet too closely can also have emotional fallout. It puts you and your child on opposite sides in a battle. You become the "food police." And like the natural little rebels that they are, kids rise to the challenge. Arguments over food will strain your relationship with your child just when you most need to stand united in dealing with diabetes. There is a better way. And that is for everyone involved to know and follow his or her job description.

The Parents' Job Description

In feeding your children, you are responsible for just four things. Parents should:

1. Get the right foods on the table. The right foods are the kinds you want the kids to eat. Choose a variety of healthful foods (*see Chapter 3 for details*). Prepare foods or buy them prepared. Let the kids help if they're old enough. If they cut the carrots themselves, they'll be more likely to eat them.

Get those good foods onto the table or into the lunch box with a minimum of fuss. Too much hype over the more healthful choices will just make kids suspicious. After all, no one gives them a PR job for things like french fries and brownies.

Away from home, children will have lots of less healthful choices, especially as they get older. But being offered mostly healthful foods at home from a young age will help your child come to actually prefer those better choices over time. He won't always make the healthiest choice—do you?—but he'll make more good choices than he would if you hadn't exposed him to good foods to begin with.

2. Make family meals frequent, peaceful, and important. Have regularly scheduled meals where family members are expected to show up and everyone is allowed to eat as much as they want of what's offered. Frequent family meals help kids meet their high nutritional needs. This can become even more important when diabetes enters the picture, depending on the insulin regimen.

Today, more and more families are eating separately, on the fly, instead of sitting down to meals together. Try to fight the trend. We know that eating every meal together is an unrealistic goal for most families. Individual schedules and responsibilities can make family meals difficult. But do the best you can. It's important.

At the dinner table, children learn not only what to eat but also how to eat it. Using table manners, managing a knife and fork, knowing how to act when faced with a new or disliked food—these are important social skills. Eating alone in front of the TV or out of a box does not produce a socially competent person. Children need to learn table manners and food preferences from you—otherwise, they'll pick them up from the other second graders in the cafeteria or from the TV. The best way we know to shape children's tastes and manners in the direction parents prefer is to eat together regularly.

Another problem occurs when mealtimes are used to argue, criticize, or hash out major conflicts. The result is indigestion and a lot of negative associations around food and eating. Catch up on everybody's news. Hand out praise. Plan for the weekend. But keep mealtimes pleasant, so everyone can eat in peace.

3. Eat what you want your children to eat. Eating what you want your children to eat is a challenge for many parents, but it eliminates a lot of problems. Children learn their eating habits the way they learn language, values, and much more: by observation. "Do as I say, not as I do" isn't nearly as effective as, "This is the way we do it in our family."

Healthy eating for your child with diabetes is the same as it is for all members of the family. And current attitudes about sweets and diabetes make it easier than you think for everyone in the family to be on the same nutritional wavelength.

Try not to single out your child with diabetes for what will surely be seen as the "punishment" of eating a variety of healthful foods while parents, brothers, or sisters eat differently. It is bound to create problems and resentments.

Instead, use diabetes as an opportunity to improve everyone's nutrition. Good food is the cornerstone of good health. Eating well fuels an active life and keeps illness to a minimum. It provides energy and gives you healthy skin and hair. It reduces risk for cancer, osteoporosis, and heart disease. These are not benefits that should be reserved only for the family member with diabetes. Everyone benefits from a sensible approach to fat in the diet. No one should be eating too many sweets.

4. Set the rules and then stay in charge! You choose and prepare the food, and you set the mealtime rules. Sometimes, children will question those choices and challenge the rules. That's expected. When it happens, stick by your guns with as much calm as you can muster. Children need to know what to expect. Be firm and consistent. It's not helpful to the family, to the child, or even to ongoing diabetes control to let short-term concerns about blood sugar disrupt the reassuring and predictable flow of family love or discipline.

The Child's Job Description

When it comes to eating, children are responsible for two things. They should:

1. Decide how much to eat of the available foods. Have faith. Children don't voluntarily starve themselves. When they're hungry, they eat. And what's more, if left to their own devices, most children even eat the right amount for their needs.

2. Follow family rules for mealtime behavior. Part of your job as a parent is making sure that mealtimes are pleasant for everyone—you included. This means that you will have expectations or rules about how everyone behaves at the table. These rules will include things like sitting in your chair while you're eating, not throwing food, not yelling. The particulars will depend on your own style and on your children's ages. Are your family meals casual, or do you "dress" for dinner? Are fingers acceptable utensils, or is everyone over the age of two expected to use a knife and fork? Whatever your rules are, the children need to follow them. When they don't do so after a couple of reminders, it's okay to ask them, firmly and calmly, to leave the table so everyone else can eat in peace. Not setting and enforcing rules may make it easier for children to use their diabetes to manipulate you and the rest of the family.

We know that this system can sound frightening to the parents of a child with diabetes, but it's the best approach we know. And it does work. It is possible to keep your child with diabetes safe and shape her lifetime eating habits without creating major power struggles over food. You may win a battle or two when you try to micromanage your child's eating, but you are in a war that cannot be won. If you're interested in avoiding food battles and in helping your children learn to choose foods wisely and control their own diets for a lifetime, follow the parent and child job descriptions given above.

THE BOTTOM LINE

Forcing children to eat doesn't work, nor does withholding food from hungry kids. To avoid fights and help children develop internal control over eating, follow the job descriptions:

The Parents' Job Description

1. Get the right foods on the table.
2. Make family meals frequent, peaceful, and important.
3. Eat what you want your children to eat.
4. Set the rules and then stay in charge!

The Child's Job Description

1. Decide how much to eat of the available foods.
2. Follow family rules for mealtime behavior.

2

How to Tell if He's Eating the Right Amount

Brandon was about average height for a three-year-old and as solid as a brick wall. He was a living study in perpetual motion. He didn't just walk, he trotted or ran. He didn't just hug you when he burst through the office door, he launched himself straight into your arms. His dad pronounced him to be "all boy and a yard wide," which seemed an understatement to us all.

He was obviously thriving, but his eating was worrying his mother. "How can he eat so much?" she asked. "The dietitian gave us a 1,200-calorie meal plan, but he's never satisfied with that. He gets angry when I won't let him have another piece of bread or more cereal. When I tell him he has to wait until snack time, he throws a fit. I try to fill him up with carrot and celery sticks, but he's back demanding more in no time. He can't go on eating twice as much as other three-year-olds and not turn into a butterball!"

It looked to us like Brandon probably needed exactly what his body was telling him

We suspected that if Mom stopped trying to limit his eating, he wouldn't be quite so desperate about it.

to eat. We suggested a trial of putting the food on the table, letting Brandon eat as much as he liked, and keeping track of it all. We would help with insulin adjustments over the phone, if necessary. But we wanted to see exactly what Brandon's appetite urged him to eat. We were pretty sure that his weight wouldn't be a problem and that his diabetes control could be worked around his very healthy appetite. We also suspected that if Mom stopped trying to limit his eating, he wouldn't be quite so desperate about it. All of that proved to be true.

Learning to Trust Your Child's Appetite

Over the years, we have suggested to many parents that they stop trying to control how much their children eat. It's seldom a popular suggestion. Some of these folks have been pressuring their children to eat ever since they first coaxed a nipple into their baby's mouth. Others have been withholding food. Like Brandon's mom, they think they and the doctor know better than the child does how much he should eat. The prospect of sitting back and letting nature take its course makes them nervous. Those in the first group worry that if they stopped urging their children to eat, the kids would not eat at all. The others were sure that their kids, if left alone, would never stop eating.

Such things seldom happen. True eating disorders (*see Chapter 9*) exist, but they are the exception rather than the rule. Normally, the body adjusts appetite to actual energy needs extremely well.

So how is the appetite-regulating system supposed to work? Under normal conditions, people eat when they're hungry and stop when they're full. The amount of food that their own body tells them to eat is the right amount to maintain their natural body type, whether it is average or heavy, muscular or slim. Although the system can be side-tracked by certain conditions, when everything's operating as it should, appetite is well-tuned to calorie needs.

You can look to nature to see how this system should work before you try it. To begin with, obesity almost never exists in animals living in the wild. Even when the African veldt is teeming with antelope, lions maintain a normal lion weight. They eat to satisfy their hunger. When they're not hungry, they lie around in the shade, explore the territory, teach the kids how to stalk, and generally live the good life.

At the other end of the spectrum, starvation is virtually never self-imposed in animals. In the animal kingdom, starvation is only seen when there isn't enough food available. Deer starve in a drought year because their food supply disappears, not because Mother Deer didn't urge Bambi to eat more leaves. Human beings can and do operate by this same system. For most of us, hunger is the best guide to how much food to eat. Satisfaction tells us when we've had enough.

Some Things Can Confuse Normal Appetite

Nature's system sometimes breaks down when people are inactive, which is a major factor in the rise in obesity that has taken place in recent years. Our bodies weren't designed to be plopped down for hours a day in front of a TV or computer screen. Our ancestors had to be physically active to survive, so our bodies are suited to that lifestyle. When we're not active, things get out of balance. We gain weight, and our appetite gets out of sync with our energy needs. We then try to control with willpower what should be internally regulated. But that doesn't work very well, as evidenced by our huge and largely ineffective (but highly profitable) weight-loss industry. If you can get your kids up off the couch and onto their bikes or the playground, you greatly increase the chances that their appetite will match their energy needs.

Another situation that can get in the way of normal appetite control is the "super-size" phenomenon. Eating out, especially in fast food restaurants, has become more common. But parents need to exert some control when the family is eating out, just as they choose what goes on the table at home. One step is to help kids choose the size of menu items that's appropriate for their age. "Super-sizing" is tempting—for just a little more money, you can get as much as three times more food (and calories). It's easy to overindulge, especially since there aren't other items to fill out the meal. At home, you may have raw vegetables, salad, another slice of meat, or fruit to fill in the niches of appetite. In the car on the way to soccer, all you've got is what's in the bag.

What All This Means for Children with Diabetes

Maybe you're thinking that this is all very well and good for other kids, but that diabetes changes the rules. While it's true that there are many things diabetes changes, energy needs is not one of them. To put it another way, diabetes doesn't affect how much food your child needs. Energy needs depend on body size, growth, metabolic rate, activity level (a big factor in Brandon's case), and other factors. They also vary a lot from child to child and even from day to day in the same child. The trick is to help the child with diabetes eat the right amount and then provide the right amount of insulin to match it.

The reliability of our internal systems for regulating eating is now well recognized by scientists, even for children with diabetes. Unfortunately, not all healthcare providers are aware of it yet. For a long time, children with diabetes received prescribed meal plans. The amount of food the child was to eat was set, just like the insulin dose, usually by the doctor or dietitian, based on the child's body weight. He consulted a chart or punched a few numbers into a calculator and said, "1,500 calories," or some other nice, round number. The child with diabetes was then expected to eat just that much every day: no more, no less.

Those calculated calorie levels were almost never exactly right, and often they were way off base. It's not easy to accurately predict someone's calorie needs. Body size is only one factor. Activity level and metabolic rate are also extremely important. For example, researchers have shown that big, heavy babies actually eat less (on average) than small, wiry infants who tend to be more active. Are heavy babies less active because they're heavy, or are they heavy because they're inactive? Maybe they're heavy and inactive because it's their nature. No one knows for sure. But we do know that there's no way to precisely predict a given person's energy (or calorie) needs. However, when our appetite is regulated naturally, it is extremely precise and adjusts automatically for growth and activity. The body can be more exact than any dietitian with a calculator.

Start with Usual Eating Habits

Calculating a prescribed calorie level is no longer considered the best way to design a meal plan for type 1 diabetes. Today, the American Diabetes Association directs healthcare providers to base nutrition advice on an assessment of each person's "usual eating habits" and then match the insulin to that pattern. This guideline recognizes each person's internal system for regulating appetite and weight. If your child's weight is already in the desirable range, then he's been eating the right amount. It makes much more sense to find out what that amount is and then base his diabetes meal plan (if one will be used) and insulin doses on that rather than starting with a predetermined plan that may not be right. If your child's weight is above or below the desirable range, his activity and eating habits need to be reviewed to see if there is a problem.

Ideally, the diabetes management plan should incorporate the child's existing eating pattern as well as the family's actual schedule, lifestyle, and food preferences. That's the best way to ensure that the family and the child will be able to manage the plan successfully.

To make this approach work, the dietitian will ask you to keep good records of what your child eats and drinks for a period of three days to a week or more. The dietitian will analyze those records to determine the usual number of calories and amount of carbohydrate eaten and the typical pattern of meals and snacks. A basic meal plan is then drawn up that translates this pattern into a particular meal planning system, such as carbohydrate counting or exchanges (*for more on this, see Chapter 4*). Your child's insulin regimen—types of insulin, number of injections, dose amounts, and timing—should closely match his typical menu. The results of your child's blood sugar tests should then be used to refine the match between food and insulin.

Table 2.1 shows how Lucy's (*see Chapter 1*) usual eating pattern was translated into a meal plan that counts carbohydrate. Notice that the dietitian didn't change Lucy's typical menu. She just translated what Lucy ate into grams of carbohydrate to help Mom and Dad manage the insulin-balancing act.

Knowing what your child eats in terms of grams of carbohydrate, exchanges, or calories enables you to make appropriate adjustments if, for example, your child is unusually hungry or if your selection of foods is limited. Depending on the situation and your own approach, you might adjust the insulin dose, substitute a different food, or encourage more or less activity to keep insulin doses in tune with the situation. Such adjustments can be useful in keeping blood sugar under control when life isn't.

Is He Eating Enough?

There are two easy-to-check results that tell you whether your child is getting the right amount of food. One is a short-term test, and the other takes a longer view.

TABLE 2.1 **Carbohydrate Counting Meal Plan Based on Usual Intake**

	Lucy's Food Record	Carbohydrate Count Meal Plan	
Meal or Snack	Food Eaten and Amount	Carbohydrate/ Item g	Total Carbohydrate g
Breakfast	1/2 cup milk	6	
	1/4 cup rice baby cereal	10	
	1/3 cup orange juice	10	
	1 scrambled egg	0	~25
Morning Snack	1/3 cup milk	4	
	1 zwieback	5	~10
Lunch	1/2 cup milk	6	
	1/3 slice wheat toast with	5	
	2 tsp. peanut butter	0	
	1/4 ripe banana	8	~20
Afternoon Snack	1/2 cup milk	6	
	2 arrowroot cookies	9	~15
Dinner	1/2 cup milk	6	
	1/4 cup oat baby cereal	10	
	1 soda cracker	3	
	2 tbs. cooked carrots	2	
	2 tbs. applesauce	4	~25
Bedtime Snack	1/3 cup milk	4	
	1 zwieback	5	
	2 baby sausages	0	~10

Hunger Is the Best Short-Term Measure

If your child is hungry all the time, chances are good that he's just not getting enough to eat. Hunger usually reflects a true need for energy, so if your child is constantly hungry, talk to your healthcare team. Don't try to "tough it out" on your own. Withholding food from a hungry child is neither necessary nor helpful, and it's hard on everyone. If it becomes a pattern, it can make the child desperate and obsessive about food. The meal plan, if your child has a set one, may need adjusting. Or the insulin plan may need to be reexamined so that your child can eat what he needs and get the food value from everything he eats. Keep in mind that it is normal for appetite to vary from day to day—

sometimes by quite a lot. These variations can be even more pronounced when a child goes in to or out of a growth spurt.

Growth Is the Best Long-Term Measure

Children grow normally only if their nutritional needs are being met. Your child's medical chart probably contains a growth grid, such as the ones shown in Figures 2.1 and 2.2 (*see Chapter 10 for infant charts*). These grids are based on the growth patterns of thousands of normally growing children. They make it possible to track your child's height and weight, watching for any changes from his usual pattern as well as comparing it to the average. You have a right to see and discuss the growth grid with your doctor or dietitian at your child's visits.

You'll notice that the grids have a series of curved lines already drawn in. Reading from the lowest line to the highest, the lines are labeled with the numbers 5, 10, and so on, through 95. These numbers are percentiles. The percentile number tells what percentage of the whole population of children who are growing normally at a given age were lighter or shorter than the number that falls on the line. The doctor, nurse, or dietitian enters your child's height and weight on the appropriate grid at each visit. In a medical version of "connect the dots," these values reveal a curved line that represents your child's growth pattern.

For example, the growth grid for eight-year-old Josh, discussed in the Introduction, is shown in Figure 2.3. Josh's growth pattern for height had been around the 60th percentile since he was a baby, which means that about 60 percent of kids were shorter than Josh at each age, and about 40 percent were taller. His growth slowed around the time his diabetes was diagnosed. That's common. He was running out of insulin and couldn't grow properly. With treatment, things improved and his growth got back on track. However, his growth slowed again when his diabetes was in poor control and he had outgrown his old meal plan.

Notice that the grids include a space to fill in Mom's and Dad's stature, or height. This gives the healthcare team a reference point for judging whether a child is probably growing to his or her potential. Say Dad is a forward for the NBA and Mom can wash the top of the mini-van without a stepstool, but their three-year-old's height is at the 15th percentile. The doctor would probably watch that child's growth and nutrition habits closely because the pattern would be unexpected

BOYS: 2 TO 18 YEARS
PHYSICAL GROWTH
NCHS PERCENTILES*

NAME_____ RECORD #_____

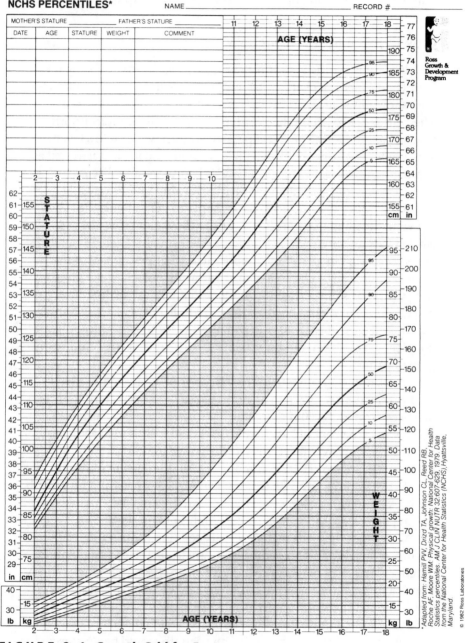

*Adapted from: Hamill PVV, Drizd TA, Johnson CL, Reed RB, Roche AF, Moore WM. Physical growth: National Center for Health Statistics percentiles. AM J CLIN NUTR 32:607-629, 1979. Data from the National Center for Health Statistics (NCHS), Hyattsville, Maryland.

© 1982 Ross Laboratories

Ross Growth & Development Program

FIGURE 2.1 Growth Grid for Boys

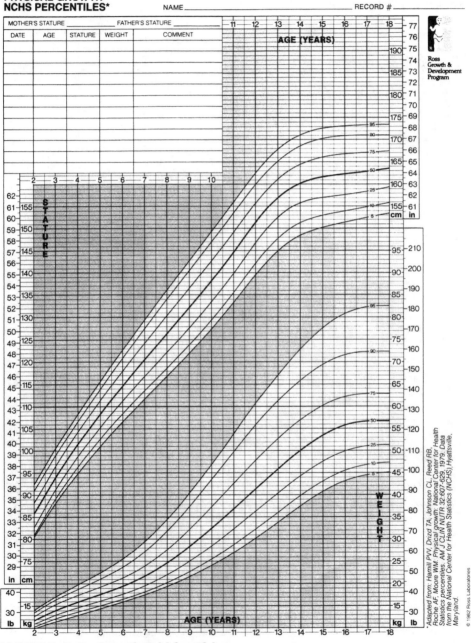

GIRLS: 2 TO 18 YEARS
PHYSICAL GROWTH
NCHS PERCENTILES*

FIGURE 2.2 Growth Grid for Girls

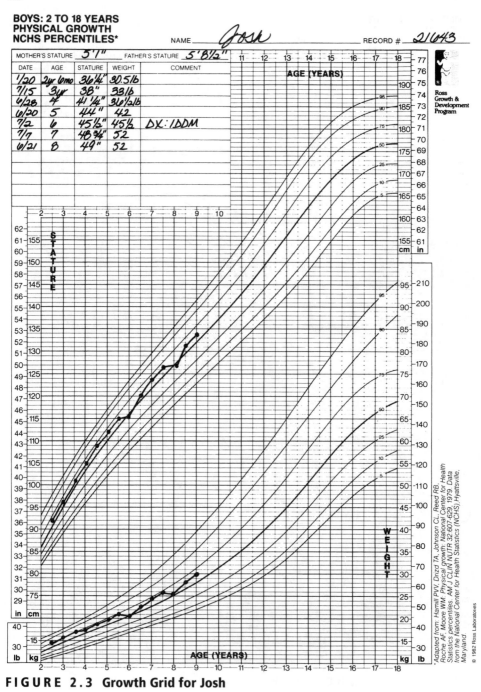

BOYS: 2 TO 18 YEARS
PHYSICAL GROWTH
NCHS PERCENTILES*

NAME _Josh_   RECORD # _21643_

MOTHER'S STATURE _5'7"_   FATHER'S STATURE _5'8½"_

DATE	AGE	STATURE	WEIGHT	COMMENT
1/20	2yr 6mo	36¼"	30.5lb	
7/15	3yr	38"	38lb	
6/28	4	41¼"	36½lb	
6/20	5	44"	42	
7/2	6	45½"	45½	DX: IDDM
7/7	7	48¾"	52	
6/21	8	49"	52	

*Adapted from: Hamill PVV, Drizd TA, Johnson CL, Reed RB, Roche AF, Moore WM. Physical growth: National Center for Health Statistics percentiles. AM J CLIN NUTR 32:607-629, 1979. Data from the National Center for Health Statistics (NCHS), Hyattsville, Maryland.

© 1982 Ross Laboratories

Ross
Growth &
Development
Program

F I G U R E 2.3 Growth Grid for Josh

in the child of such tall parents. However, if Dad is a jockey and Mom sits on a pillow to see over the dashboard of the car, the 15th percentile is expected.

Keeping diabetes in control by matching insulin to the right amount of food eaten allows a child to fulfill his or her genetic potential. A child's growth potential is often similar to that of one or both parents or other family members. Occasionally, a child gets a blueprint like Uncle Mort (the only tall man in an otherwise short family) or Grandma Ellen (the only tiny, fine-boned person in a family of muscular, outdoorsy folks). If your child seems to be following a different pattern than the rest of the family, it may take a while to figure out what his pattern is supposed to be. Each person's adult height and weight are reached according to a fairly predictable pattern of growth. That pattern can be followed from infancy through the teenage years using the growth grids.

Another important piece of information that can be obtained from the growth grid is a quick check of the relationship between height and weight. In spite of expectations created by the use of emaciated young girls and women to advertise everything from hiking boots to kitchen products, people *do* come in different sizes and body types: thin, muscular, average, and heavy. For example, a girl with a muscular build might consistently follow a weight curve at the 70th percentile and a height at a somewhat lower percentile, say, the 60th. Or a boy with a slim build might consistently have a weight curve that hovers around the 50th percentile with a height curve a bit higher, perhaps at the 60th. The height and weight of a child with an average build would tend to fall at about the same percentile rank.

If there is a change in this established relationship, it's time for some detective work. For example, Julie had always been on the slim side, with a height around the 60th percentile and a weight around the 50th percentile. Over a six-month period when she was nine years old, her weight quickly moved up to the 65th percentile while her height stayed at around the 60th percentile. Even though Julie wasn't actually heavy, the pattern was unusual for her. It alerted her doctor to ask if she had experienced an increase in hypoglycemia (and ate extra food to treat it) and to check her insulin doses.

In monitoring your child's growth, the important questions to ask the doctor, nurse, or dietitian are:

- Do my child's percentile rankings for height and weight make sense for a member of our family?
- Is he staying on his growth curve?
- Is the relationship between the height and weight percentiles appropriate and staying about the same?

If the answer to all of these questions is yes, then your child is eating the right amount of food. You can feel confident of this even if he's eating a lot less than his brother did at the same age or twice as much as the other third graders. However, if the answer to any of these questions is no, his eating, activity level, diabetes management, and general health need to be closely checked to find out why.

Food and Insulin Balance Is Essential

To manage diabetes in kids:

- They should eat the amount of food they need.
- The right amount of insulin should be given at the right time to allow their bodies to use the foods they eat.

It sounds easy, but it's not.

Most children with diabetes need about 3/10 to 4/10 of a unit of insulin for every pound of body weight. Many kids need less during the temporary "honeymoon" that often follows diagnosis and need more during adolescence, when hormones can increase insulin needs dramatically.

Here's an example of a fairly average youngster. A 60-pound child will probably be on a total daily insulin dose (the total of all insulins taken in a 24-hour period) of between about 18 units (60 lb. × 0.3 unit/lb.) and 24 units (60 lb. × 0.4 unit/lb.). Keep in mind, however, that everyone is different. The best way to judge your child's insulin dose is by how she's doing, not by some average calculated number. The amount of food being consumed and the total insulin dose are probably correct, even if her insulin dose is higher or lower than this average range, as long as she is:

- Experiencing reasonable blood sugar control
- Growing normally

- Active and energetic
- Not gaining or losing weight inappropriately
- Not routinely complaining of hunger

Blood sugar control may not be exactly where you want it to be, but good growth and the absence of unusual hunger tell you that the big pieces of the plan are in place.

On the other hand, ask the healthcare team to review her insulin doses and menu with you so you can figure out how to improve things if she is:

- Growing poorly
- Gaining excess weight or losing weight unintentionally
- Frequently having positive tests for urine ketones
- Frequently having high or low blood sugars
- Generally experiencing poor blood sugar control

Effects of Poor Diabetes Control

A healthy appetite and normal growth are good indicators that a child is getting enough to eat, as along as the diabetes is in reasonable control. But when blood sugar is consistently high, the picture can get confusing. Sugar and all the calories it contains flow out in the urine when the blood sugar level is fairly high (above 180 mg/dl or 10 mmol for most people). This can make it look like little George needs a lot more food than he is getting, or that he can "eat and eat and never gain an ounce." Because needed calories aren't staying in the body, his growth may slow. If the child is getting too little insulin, his body will break down fat to get the energy it needs. When he's burning fat for energy, ketones will show up in urine ketone tests. These ketones, in turn, may lessen the child's appetite. Diabetes control needs to be improved before hunger and growth will return to normal.

It can also be tough to tell how much food a child really needs when insulin doses are increased too much. Unfortunately, it's not all that rare for glucose levels to vary a lot during growth. Sometimes in our eagerness to control high blood sugars, we increase the insulin too much, which leads to low blood sugar. Then, instead of recognizing that too much insulin is being given, it's easy to be fooled into "feeding" the extra insulin to prevent and treat the lows. If this happens, the child may gain excess weight. To avoid these problems, insulin must be matched to the child's food intake, not the other way around. This is why parents need to learn how to make insulin adjustments themselves.

We hope this information has given you enough confidence to at least try out the parent and child job descriptions presented in Chapter 1. Remember, it's your job to get the right food into the house and on the table, and it's your child's job to decide what he will eat of what's available.

THE BOTTOM LINE

In all kids, including those with diabetes:

1. Appetite is usually a good indicator of actual energy needs.
2. Energy needs depend on several factors, including age, growth, size, and activity.
3. Hunger is the best short-term measure of correct calorie intake.
4. Growth is the best long-term measure of correct calorie intake.

In children with diabetes:

1. Glucose control lets the body use the energy and nutrients in food so the child can grow normally.

Jody loves carrots, but giving her other vegetables is a waste . . .

3

How to Tell if She's Eating the Right Things

Jody's mother was worried about the four-year-old's limited diet. "There are so many things on the exchange lists that she should be eating. But she just doesn't like many foods. The only cooked vegetable she'll eat is carrots. She actually gags when I give her broccoli. And what about bread? All she wants to eat is white bread or hamburger buns. Isn't she going to get sick if she doesn't start eating wheat bread pretty soon?"

When the dietitian learned a bit more about what Jody was eating, she was able to reassure her mother that the little girl was not in any immediate danger of malnutrition. Her preferred diet *was* pretty simple, even boring from an adult viewpoint. But it was also reasonably complete. People need certain nutrients, not certain foods. Jody was getting enough of the right kinds of foods to provide the nutrients she needed. Eventually, her tastes expanded, and she began to enjoy darker breads and the wide variety of vegetables,

She actually gags when I give her broccoli.

salads, and dried beans that her parents ate. But it took quite a bit of time and patience before her tastes changed.

Mom and Dad just kept putting a variety of foods on the table and eating them themselves. They gave Jody lots of choices and frequent chances to try new things without pressure. The foods she liked were there for her to choose from as well. At age four, she simply preferred plain chicken or hamburger, cooked carrots, a few raw fruits and vegetables, white bread, Cheerios, and milk. She ate those things with pleasure, but she was very suspicious of foods with coarser textures and stronger flavors.

It's fine for a youngster like Jody to eat virtually the same thing for dinner night after night, as long as the meal is nutritious and preparing it is not a burden. (If the diet is quite limited, a children's vitamin and mineral supplement can help for a time.) Forcing foods on a child almost guarantees that there will be food battles. And it violates your job description.

Still, Jody's mom was right to be concerned. We all need certain raw materials—protein, around 50 different vitamins and minerals, and a certain amount of energy—to make a healthy human body.

One Healthy Diet for One Healthy Family

As far as we know, well-controlled diabetes does not change nutritional needs, so the same foods that are good for everyone else in the family are also good for the child with diabetes. All family members will feel and perform better and have the best chance for good health if they eat well. With *uncontrolled* diabetes, the body may need even more good foods. When blood sugars are high, a large volume of urine is passed, causing calories and other nutrients to be lost. All the more reason for the child with diabetes to be getting most of her diet from basic, nutrient-rich foods, just like the rest of the family.

Feeding everyone the same reasonable and healthful diet can also help avoid arguments, resentments, and feelings of being deprived. Basically, there is no easy way to feed the child with diabetes differently from the rest of the family. It will certainly create more work, and it will probably lead to hurt feelings and conflict as well.

Still, every family is different, and you will need to weigh the pros and cons of the "one healthy diet for one healthy family" approach for your particular situation. There are several benefits. As we've said, better health for everyone and less time preparing family meals are important factors. But also consider that this approach places less pressure on the child with diabetes. There aren't so many "no's" in the house. And there's less basis for resentment, which can occur when she sees family members eat "forbidden fruit." The most likely downside of this approach is the potential for hostility from other family members. Some may feel their freedom is being stepped on by a stronger emphasis on health in family meals.

Only you can decide what works best for your family. Talk it over. Find out how everyone feels about any changes you are planning. See if you can come to an agreement about how to handle any concerns that come up. The more changes that you're considering, the more important it is to talk it all out.

Change Food Patterns Gradually

If your family is willing to go ahead—despite reservations and doubts—experiment gradually with the new order. Let's say you'd like to try switching the whole family from whole milk to one percent milk. Consider taking a month to phase in the change. It takes time for taste buds to adjust, so try to make all your experiments long enough to take this into account. First, switch to two percent milk for at least two weeks. Then check out how the family is adjusting before taking the step down to one percent milk. Other experiments in healthy eating might involve switching from chips to pretzels or from regular to lower-fat ice cream, or not buying those chocolate kisses at all.

We strongly recommend a step-by-step approach, gradually removing or substituting foods. Also take one step at a time when adding more healthful foods to family menus. It may take several tries to find vegetables that are a hit with everybody.

What if you have a family member who just won't give up certain foods? We've had more than one mom and dad who experimented with eating their "forbidden" foods on the sly. This usually involved hiding the food and then eating it late at night while the child with diabetes was sleeping. Sure, this has worked for some families, but it's not an approach that we recommend. There's a real risk for anger and hurt feelings if your child discovers your empty Dove Bar wrapper in the trash one morning. Making the enjoyment of certain foods into a clandestine operation often backfires. It can give tremendous emotional power to the very foods you want your kids to eat less often. Instead, consider occasional treats an important joy of life. Diabetes doesn't change this.

In the end, however, every family has to find its own way. Your final strategy will probably be a combination of eliminating some foods, limiting others, and substituting for still others until you have a healthier, but hopefully not totally indulgence-free, menu that the whole family can enjoy.

Although family members can all eat the same foods, we do need to keep track of how much and when the child with diabetes eats. This is the cornerstone of managing the food-insulin-exercise balancing act. But *what* is eaten can be the same for all.

How Did Nutrition Get So Complicated?

Throughout most of our history, eating did not require much thought. Tradition and simple availability determined what people ate, and this is still true in nonindustrialized societies today. In the United States and other developed countries, however, choosing healthful foods is not so easy. We now have such a huge variety of foods from which to choose that we really have to use our heads, and not just our taste buds, in deciding what to eat.

The Wisdom of Traditional Cultures

For thousands of years, the people of a given region, culture, or religion all ate essentially the same foods. The "foodways," or diet, of each culture evolved to include a mix of foods from the local area that kept people healthy. The technology to transport foods long distances didn't exist, and those who were able to choose well from the available mix were strong, powerful, and able to reproduce. Perhaps others noticed what these healthy people ate and incorporated those foods into their own diets.

For example, even though no one knew what calcium was until fairly recently, every traditional diet provided it. Cultures that kept cows or goats typically got their calcium from milk. But in other places, where adults never drank milk, there were other sources. For societies that ate ground grains, such as corn, the grinding stone often added the needed calcium. People from fishing cultures ate calcium-rich fish bones. The same is true for all the essential nutrients. Iron can come from meat, leafy vegetables, blood, and even cooking pots. Asians get most of their protein from fish, pork, soybeans, and eggs, while the major sources of protein in India are lentils, grains, and yogurt.

Every traditional diet includes sources for all the essential nutrients. Now, with nothing but advertising, our taste buds, and our ability to pay to guide us, we can make some pretty awful choices. The dramatic increase in obesity and the rising tide of heart disease and other chronic conditions make the results of our choices very clear.

The Challenge in Easy Availability

Most of us in the West get enough food today. But that wasn't always the case, and it is still not true in many places in the world. Before the mass production and shipping of food, just getting enough to eat was a full-time job, and it was hard work. You had to hunt it, grow it, or gather it from the countryside. Then you had to skin it, clean it, chop it, and build a fire to cook it. Surpluses were carefully preserved and then eaten a bit at a time, not wiped out in one Saturday night food orgy.

Compare our situation today. Fast-food restaurants are everywhere. Take-out delicacies are only as far away as your phone. Huge bags of chips wait in the pantry for a little light grazing at the end of the day. And triple fudge ripple ice cream calls your name from the freezer. It's all so easy, and it tastes so good! Most of us can get whatever we want at a fairly reasonable cost. Between easy access and the powerful influence of advertising, most people in the United States today eat a wide variety of foods.

Few people still eat the traditional foods of their ancestors. And when they do, it's often the foods for special celebrations and holidays, not the common, everyday things that guaranteed good nutrition. For example, many baked goods and sweets take a long time to prepare, so they showed up on the table infrequently, mostly at special occasions. Now someone else has done all the work, you can get them whenever you want, and they're relatively inexpensive. It takes a conscious effort, and sometimes even costs more, to pick whole grain cereal over a donut. Today we have lots of choices, many of which are nutritionally unsound. So we need to choose well to fulfill the first part of our job description: Get the right stuff on the table.

A Simple Guide to Good Nutrition

Thankfully, there's an uncomplicated tool you can use to help plan healthful meals for the whole family. It's called the Food Guide Pyramid. You've probably seen it printed on cereal boxes and bread wrappers. The American Diabetes Association and the American Dietetic Association adapted this pyramid into a Diabetes Food Pyramid.

The Diabetes Food Pyramid, shown in Figure 3.1, divides foods into six groups, because no one food contains all the needed nutrients. (Human breast milk is an exception, but it is adequate only for infants.) We know, however, that certain nutrients are found in particular kinds of foods. For example, calcium is found in all dairy products, and vitamin C is found in fruits and vegetables. If we eat from all the right groups, we get what we need without having to eat the same foods day after day.

Each Section Provides Certain Nutrients

The pyramid shows the types of food and the relative amount of each group that we need to eat each day. It also shows the number of servings needed for adequate nutrition. Table 3.1 shows how serving sizes change as a child ages.

- Grains, beans, and starchy vegetables make up the largest section of the pyramid, just as they should make up the largest portion of the diet. They are the backbone of a healthy eating plan and should be a major source of energy (or calories). They provide essential B vitamins and iron, and if you choose whole-grain varieties, they are also a good source of fiber, trace minerals (like chromium and copper), and certain plant chemicals that improve resistance to disease.
- Fruits and vegetables make up the next level of the pyramid. They are important sources of several vitamins, especially vitamins A and C, and many minerals, including trace elements. Make at least one choice high in vitamin A (from foods like carrots, dried apricots, cantaloupe, dark greens, and sweet potatoes) and another high in vitamin C (from foods like broccoli, oranges, peppers, cabbage, and strawberries). Fruits and vegetables are important sources of antioxidants and other nutrients that increase immunity and reduce risk for cancer and heart disease.

FATS

A sample adult serving is 1/8 avocado; 1 tablespoon of cream cheese or salad dressing; 1 teaspoon of margarine, oil, or mayonnaise; or 10 peanuts

SWEETS

A sample adult serving is 1/2 cup ice cream; 1 small cupcake; or 2 small cookies

ALCOHOL

If you choose to drink alcohol, limit the amount and have it with a meal. Talk to your doctor about a safe amount for you.

MEAT AND OTHER PROTEINS

(2–3 servings)

A sample adult serving is 2–3 oz. cooked lean meat, poultry, or fish; 1/2 to 3/4 cup tuna or cottage cheese; 1 egg; or 2 tablespoons peanut butter

FRUITS

(3–4 servings)

A sample adult serving is 1 small fresh fruit; 1/2 cup canned fruit; 1/4 cup dried fruit; or 1/2 cup fruit juice

MILK

(2–3 servings)

A sample adult serving is 1 cup of milk or 1 cup of yogurt

VEGETABLES

(3–5 servings)

A sample adult serving is 1/2 cup tomato or vegetable juice; 1/2 cup cooked vegetables; or 1 cup raw vegetables

GRAINS, BEANS, AND STARCHY VEGETABLES

(6 or more servings)

A sample adult serving is 1 slice of bread; 1 English muffin; 4–6 crackers; 1/2 cup cooked pasta, rice, beans, or corn; 3/4 cup dry cereal; or 1 small potato

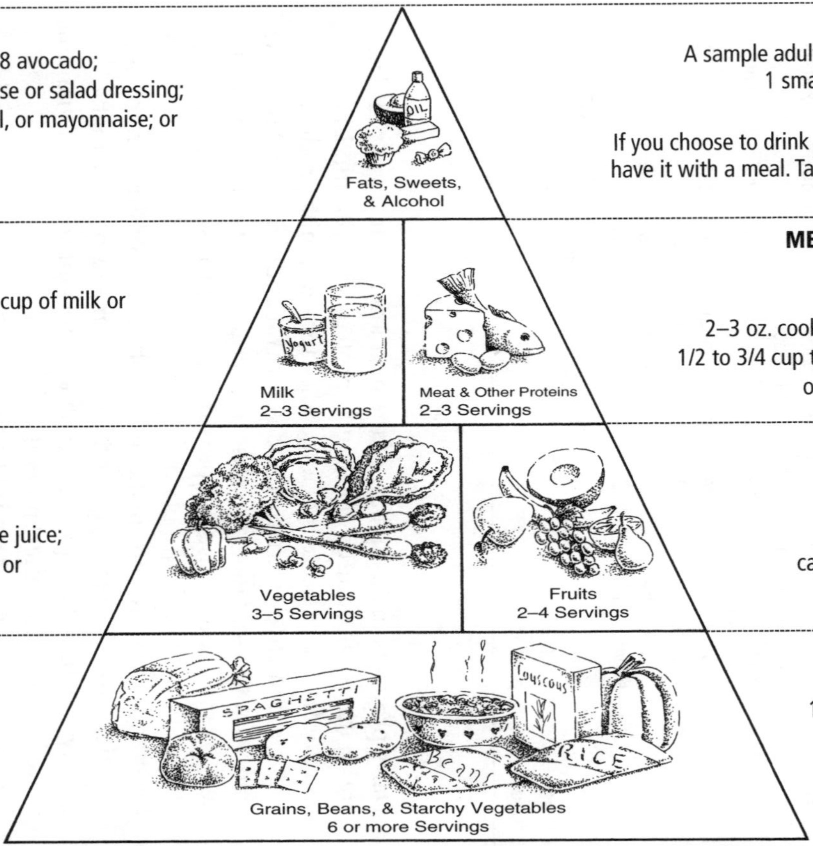

Fats, Sweets, & Alcohol

Milk
2–3 Servings

Meat & Other Proteins
2–3 Servings

Vegetables
3–5 Servings

Fruits
2–4 Servings

Grains, Beans, & Starchy Vegetables
6 or more Servings

DIABETES FOOD PYRAMID

American Diabetes Association/The American Dietetic Association

FIGURE 3.1

TABLE 3.1 Minimal Daily Nutrition Requirements: Portion Sizes Change with Age

Food Group	Infant	Toddler & Preschooler	School Age	Teen
Milk	16–24 oz.	2 cups (no more than 3 cups)	2–3 cups	4 cups
Breads/ Cereals	4 servings, about 1–2 Tbsp. or 1/4 the adult serving each	4 servings, about 1 Tbsp. per year of age or 1/4 the adult serving each	4 adult or exchange-size servings	4 adult or exchange-size servings
Fruits/ Vegetables	4–5 servings, 1–2 Tbsp. or 1/4 the adult serving each	4–5 servings, about 1 Tbsp. per year of age or 1/4 the adult serving each	4–5 adult or exchange-size servings	4–5 adult or exchange-size servings
Meat/ Protein	2 ~1/2 oz. portions	2–3 oz.	2–3 oz.	4–5 oz.

■ Dairy products make up part of the next level of the pyramid. They are an important source of calcium, protein, and vitamin D. Low- and nonfat varieties are the best choice for fluid milk products, yogurts, and cheeses once a child is past the toddler stage. For those who want to avoid dairy because of allergies or other reasons, fortified soy milk and cheese can provide many of the same nutrients, plus additional healthful plant chemicals.

■ Meat and other proteins make up the other part of the third pyramid tier. Fish, chicken, eggs, and lower-fat meats provide high-quality protein. Many proteins can be important sources of vitamins as well as iron and other minerals.

■ Sweets and fats are shown in the tiny top portion of the pyramid. These foods are a source of extra calories (and pleasure) once basic needs are met, but if eaten in large amounts, they can keep us from eating the things we need for complete nutrition. Fats include those added in cooking or at the table as well as those found naturally in some foods. Eating according to the pyramid means limiting sweets, fried foods, gravies, sauces, butter, margarine, and salad dressings.

Eating the minimum number of recommended servings each day from the pyramid gives kids the minimum amounts of protein, vitamins, and minerals their bodies require. Of course, most children need to eat more than that to get the energy that their growing bodies demand, particularly if they are physically active. For older, bigger, and more active kids who need more food, the remaining calories should ideally come in the same general proportions as shown on the pyramid—in other words, more of the same. At least in the meals and snacks you offer at home, try to keep the relative proportion of fats and sweets small, compared with the amounts of starches, fruits, vegetables, proteins, and dairy foods.

How Much Soda?

Several troublesome food trends have emerged or grown stronger since the first edition of *Sweet Kids*. Fewer family meals are prepared and eaten at home, and we're relying more on fast foods and other convenience items. Another disturbing trend is that everyone, right down to the youngest child, is drinking more soda and other manufactured beverages. These items are heavily advertised, and as a result, some children drink several large sodas each day. This trend should be reversed.

Kids eat only so many calories in a day. If they are getting several hundred calories a day from soda (one 12-ounce can provides about 150 calories—and that's not even a typical super size drink), it is sure to displace more important foods.

Even diet sodas contain two things that are a big concern: All bubbly drinks contain phosphorus, and many contain caffeine. High phosphorus is bad for bones, so not only are soda drinkers weakening bones, they also are not getting enough calcium to begin with because they are not drinking milk. High phosphorus intake is particularly worrisome in kids who have replaced milk at meals with soda. Caffeine is an addictive, mood-altering substance, and its long-term use from childhood into adulthood has not been studied. Kids should avoid or limit caffeine intake and should limit their soda drinking as well.

A Note about Vegetarian Diets

Vegetarian diets are more common than they once were. There are several approaches to vegetarian eating. Some people avoid only red meat. Others avoid all types of meat and poultry. A vegetarian may also avoid animal products entirely, including milk, cheese, and eggs. People adopt a vegetarian eating style for different reasons. It may be a requirement of their religion, a response to concerns about the environment, or an ethical aversion to killing animals. Others find a vegetarian eating style more economical or healthful. And some people with diabetes follow a vegetarian diet because research suggests that vegetable protein may be easier on the kidneys than animal protein.

Regardless of the reason for it, eating a vegetarian diet is perfectly compatible with both good health and good diabetes control. Vegetarians, too, can use the Diabetes Food Pyramid as a nutritional blueprint, but the foods in the protein section will include cheese, eggs, beans, peas, lentils, tofu, and soy products, rather than meats. Total vegetarians (or vegans—those who avoid all animal products) don't eat cheese or eggs. For them, the dairy or milk group will consist of soy milk and soy cheese rather than dairy products.

Special Needs of Vegetarian Diets

Vegetarian diets that eliminate all animal products can be hard for very young children to digest. If this is the case, they may have problems getting enough calories and protein from what they eat. Vegetarian diets are much more bulky than diets that include meat, cheese, and milk. To help overcome this problem, it is probably best to include at least milk and eggs as protein sources in the diets of kids preschool age and younger. Also, adequate fat should be added in cooking and at the table to provide enough calories in the small volume of food that these very young children can eat. It is important to make sure that hard-to-digest foods—beans and cracked grains, for example—are cooked thoroughly and then mashed or chopped to help young jaws and intestinal tracts. The growth of all youngsters, especially those with diabetes, should be monitored, as this is the best indication that they're getting all the nutrients and energy they need.

Two nutrients are hard to get in vegetarian diets: iron and vitamin B_{12}. Most nutritionists and doctors recommend supplements of these nutrients for all vegetarians.

One final point regarding vegetarian diets for children with diabetes: Be aware that meat, fish, and poultry don't affect blood sugar very much, and neither do some of the vegetarian sources of protein, such as eggs, peanut butter, and cheese. Other vegetarian proteins, however, contain considerable amounts of carbohydrate, which needs to be counted when matching food and insulin. Beans, lentils, and black-eyed peas, for example, have quite a bit of carbohydrate. In fact, we included them with starches on the Diabetes Food Pyramid to make it easier to remember to count their carbohydrate value. If your child with diabetes is following a vegetarian diet, don't forget to count the carbohydrate value of the high-starch protein foods.

Real Kids' Diets and the Food Pyramid

Table 3.2 shows what a normally picky 4-year-old girl and her active 10-year-old brother each ate in one day. Both are eating according to the pyramid, but the amounts are different because Lindy and Jason differ in age, size, and activity level.

Can you tell from looking at the foods listed in Table 3.2 which of these children has diabetes? Both children are eating from all the pyramid groups, and both are eating small amounts of sweets. It's Jason who has diabetes. Lindy has pretty simple tastes, but all the types of food required for good health are there.

Is This Normal Pickiness?

What about children who have truly odd food preferences? Or unusual eating habits? How can you tell if your child's food choices are abnormal?

Normal eating varies—a lot! In fact, it varies so much that we've had a hard time coming up with a simple definition. Every time we think we've found a reasonable guideline, we think of all the exceptions to the rule. From the first time a baby is put to the breast, a unique eating personality is apparent. Food preferences, speed of eating, even the noises kids make while they eat are individual. It's hard to draw a clear line between normal and abnormal eating.

Differences in Taste Perception

Some kids seem to have unique or unusual taste preferences. Most babies and young children seem to prefer milder flavors and neutral

TABLE 3.2 What Two Real Kids Eat in a Day

Pyramid Group	Lindy, 4 years old	Jason, 10 years old
Grains, Beans, and Starchy Vegetables	3/4 cup cereal, 1 slice sandwich bread, 5 pretzels, 11 miniature graham bear cookies, 1/2 of a dinner roll	1 1/2 cups cereal, 4 slices sandwich bread, 15 pretzels, 25 miniature graham bear cookies, 1 baked potato, 2 dinner rolls, pizza crust from 1 slice
Fruits	1/2 cup apple juice, 1 fresh apricot, 1/2 cup strawberries	8 oz. apple juice, 2 apricots, 1 cup strawberries, 1 banana, 1 kiwi
Vegetables	3 carrot sticks, 1/2 cup green salad, 4 cherry tomatoes	6 carrot and celery sticks, 1 1/2 cups green salad, 4 cherry tomatoes, 2 stalks steamed broccoli, 1 can vegetable juice
Milk and Dairy Products	2 cups milk	2 cups 2% milk, 1 carton low-fat yogurt, 1 cup chocolate milk
Meat and Other Proteins	1 slice cheese, 1 slice roast beef	3 oz. string cheese, 3 Tbsp. peanut butter, 3 slices roast beef, 1 slice cheese pizza
Sweets and Fats	1 tsp. mayonnaise, 1 tsp. salad dressing, 1 tsp. margarine, 5 gummy bears	2 tsp. mayonnaise, 2 Tbsp. salad dressing, 3 tsp. margarine, 2 oz. light sour cream, 10 gummy bears

or sweet foods over things that are sour or bitter. But beyond these normal characteristics of younger palates, some kids are just "wired" for greater taste sensitivity. Remember, every adult wine taster and gourmet cook started life as a kid—probably one who drove his parents crazy at the dinner table. Keep in mind that you can't taste what your child is tasting. Their own immature taste buds, inexperienced palate, or personal degree of flavor or odor sensitivity give them a unique taste experience of any given food.

But be patient. Foods that were once accepted willingly or even demanded daily can suddenly end up on the 10 Most Hated List (and vice versa). Think of foods you once hated but eventually learned to enjoy. If you can remember how your own tastes have changed, it may help you relax a bit when your children express odd food preferences or dislikes.

Personality Is another Factor

On the personality side of picky behavior, some people are just suspicious of anything new and are slow to change. Kids with this type of personality will probably resist eating any new food. Other children are very open to new experiences of all kinds, and food is just part of that general outlook on life. You know your own child. The way she responds to food will probably just be an extension of her overall approach to life. You won't change it. The child will probably change somewhat with age and experience, but whether she does or not, keep your cool. Keep mealtimes pleasant to ensure that food is not a source of arguments. Food fights are a losing battle in any family. But they're especially harmful in the family dealing with diabetes.

When they balk at foods, remember your job description. Get a variety of the right kinds of foods on the table and eat them yourself. Set your own mealtime rules and enforce them. In your house, everyone might have to at least taste whatever is served. Maybe you're training your kids to say, "Thanks, Mom, but I don't care for more," instead of tossing a half-chewed morsel on the table and shouting, "Yuck, that's gross!" Whatever your rules are, be consistent. Apply them equally to all the kids in the family.

Evaluating Eating: What's Normal?

As far as knowing when a quirky eating preference or behavior may actually be a cause for concern, consider the following points:

- There is no food that everybody has to like and eat. It's natural to want to eat more of the foods we like and less (or none!) of the foods we dislike. As long as your child is eating some selections from all the food groups of the pyramid, she'll do fine nutritionally. As for the terminally picky, they will probably be all right in the short run if they eat some choices from each *level* of the pyramid (for example, a child who refuses all vegetables but eats fruit, or a child who won't eat meat but takes dairy products). But if your child's choices stay that limited for more than a few weeks, a dietitian should review several days of the child's meal plan to find out if this behavior is putting her at any real risk. Observe your child's growth, general health, and energy level. If they're good, then chances are excellent that eating a peanut butter sandwich for lunch every day is not causing serious problems. Food jags usually die a natural death if you don't make a big deal out of them.

■ Does your child seem to enjoy her food? If so, this is a good sign that no major problems with food exist. On the other hand, if she's tense and seems overly worried about either having or avoiding certain foods, it might be a good idea to consult with a physician, dietitian, or counselor.

■ If anything about your child's eating drives you so nuts that you can't let it slide, get some help in evaluating it. There may really be an eating problem, or you just may need some help in dealing with your child's normal quirkiness better. Either way, a pediatric dietitian or a family counselor will probably be able to help. (*See Chapter 9 for more about preventing, identifying, and treating serious eating disorders.*)

You can use the Diabetes Food Pyramid to plan nutritious and delicious meals for the whole family. Healthy eating won't eliminate enjoyment, favorite foods, or special occasions. Every food fits into the pyramid somewhere, so all can be part of a nutritious eating plan and can fit into your plan for diabetes control. Variety is important. Offer it, but relax. Children will build up their repertoire of preferred foods slowly over time. Support this process through your own healthful eating, but don't pressure your child to eat certain foods. By questioning and experimenting, you can develop a way of dealing with food that will promote good health for the whole family. That same plan can work for your child with diabetes, reducing or even eliminating many of the food-related stresses that have troubled you in the past. (*For more information on the Food Pyramid, see the resource list at the end of Chapter 4.*)

THE BOTTOM LINE

1. People need certain nutrients, not certain foods, to be healthy.
2. All foods can be included in a healthy eating plan for the child with diabetes as well as other family members.
3. Withholding sweets makes them seem more desirable. Incorporate them into meals in appropriate amounts so they can be enjoyed without displacing needed nutrients.
4. When sodas become a child's usual beverage, they compromise healthy bones. Water, milk, and fruit juice all have nutritional benefits without the negative aspects of sodas.
5. The Diabetes Food Pyramid can be the basis of both healthful family meals and diabetes food management.
6. Some kids are picky eaters, but likes and dislikes usually change with age and experience.
7. Keep getting the right stuff on the table, and kids will eventually learn to like most of it.

4

The Basics of Diabetes Nutrition

José's mother, Anna, is more than a mere survivor of the battle to help her child live well with diabetes. She is to diabetes strategy and chutzpah what General George Patton was to the 7th Army in World War II: a mover and a shaker. She has worked hard to keep her family's life and meals as normal as possible. Her thoughts about living with José's diabetes mirror those of many parents we know.

"As soon as diabetes entered the picture, food took on a larger-than-life role. It would have been so easy to lose all the joy of preparing and eating food, because we had to constantly think of things that were never an issue before: when to eat, for instance, and what the ingredients were in everything. Food is a very personal thing. A lot more than nutrition goes into choosing what we eat. But diabetes can make it seem like nothing matters but the hard facts: how big a portion? how much carbohydrate? I would be totally demoralized if someone doled out 11 Teddy Grahams to me, and I won't do it to José.

José's mother is to diabetes strategy what General Patton was to the 7th Army in World War II: a mover and a shaker.

"The way diabetes dominates family meals can make you feel like you've lost a basic freedom. And the 'foreverness' of it can be overwhelming, too. That's why it's so important not to overdo the rigid 'diet' attitude. No one can stay rigid all the time."

We couldn't agree more. Our work with families over the years has convinced us that overly rigid guidelines—"Eat exactly this, no more and no less," or "Never let your child eat that"—are unrealistic, unproductive, and, maybe most important of all, unnecessary. We believe that the more you know about nutrition, diabetes, and effective family problem solving, the more freedom you will have. With knowledge, practice, and problem solving, you can earn an impressive degree of freedom in food choices, greater meal-timing options, and enjoyable family meals free of battles. Notice that we said "earn," because these gifts don't just waltz in off the street. You work for them. But we think they're more than worth the effort.

The Basics of Nutrition and Diabetes

Why is food such an important part of every plan to manage diabetes? Because diabetes takes away the body's ability to use the energy from foods properly. And since energy is essential for life and health, restoring that ability is the major focus of treatment.

The food we eat breaks down into a form of sugar called glucose. Glucose is the body's main fuel—just as gasoline is the fuel that runs your car. When glucose from food enters the bloodstream, the body is supposed to release insulin so that glucose can enter body cells, but in people with type 1 diabetes, the insulin is not produced. Once in the cells, glucose keeps the heart beating, the muscles moving, and more.

Because your child's insulin-producing cells don't work anymore, the system can't do its job. Without effective management, insulin is not where it's supposed to be when it's supposed to be there. Glucose builds up in the bloodstream instead of going to the cells. As a result, the body is starved for energy. In addition, tissues get damaged because glucose is flooding a lot of places in the body where it's not supposed to be.

Before diabetes, your child's pancreas automatically produced the insulin his body needed. It put in short bursts of insulin when he ate: a little when he ate a small amount, and a lot when he ate more. It lowered the insulin level when he was active. It met his needs exactly. Now that system no longer works, and you're in the business of "playing pancreas." Working from the outside, you and your child try to balance food, insulin, and exercise, using blood sugar testing to guide you.

Food, especially the carbohydrate (or starch and sugar) it contains, is one of the major things that determines insulin needs. To control blood sugar, you need to know what is being eaten and how much insulin it takes to handle it. When you pull off that balancing act, blood sugar hovers somewhere near the normal range most of the time. The results are never perfect. Our tools for diabetes management don't ever work as precisely as a functioning pancreas. But we can come pretty close—close enough for your child to feel great, grow normally, and remain healthy. This chapter focuses on understanding the food and insulin part of this balancing act.

Today's Tools for Insulin Replacement

This is a very exciting time in the diabetes world. Our tools and our understanding have grown in recent years, making it possible for people to reach target blood sugars without all of the lifestyle restrictions that were once required. To get the most out of these tools, it helps to have a clear picture of how insulin works under normal conditions. Be aware that not all types of insulin have received approval for use in children—check with your child's doctor for the most up-to-date information.

The Body Closely Regulates Insulin

In people who don't have diabetes, blood sugars are maintained in a healthy range because the body regulates insulin levels according to need. Their bodies provide a low background, or "basal," level of insulin between meals and overnight. This background insulin enables the body to use stores of glucose for energy when glucose isn't coming in from food. But what about the blood sugar surges that occur after meals? The pancreases of those who don't have diabetes pump out extra insulin, in exactly the right amount, to counteract after-meal rises in blood sugar. Once this happens, the body's level of insulin falls very quickly back to the basal level. This is why people without diabetes almost never have low blood sugar reactions.

People with diabetes, however, must regulate insulin doses themselves. NPH, insulin glargine (Lantus), Lente, and Ultralente are the insulins given most often by pen or syringe to meet these basal needs. When an insulin pump is used, rapid-acting insulin is given continuously in very small amounts for the same purpose.

The rapid-acting insulins (Novolog and Humalog) act most like the insulin the body produces to counteract after-meal blood sugar surges. These "bolus" doses of insulin are our best option for meal coverage, whether they are given by pen, pump, or syringe. These insulins peak quickly and disappear in about three hours.

Regular [R] insulin acts much longer. It peaks two or more hours after it's taken and can remain in the body for six to eight hours. When it is used to cover a meal, a snack must be eaten a few hours later to prevent low blood sugars. Similarly, when NPH or Lente are given in the morning to cover lunch, snacks are usually needed in the morning and afternoon because these insulins keep basal insulin levels too high between meals. Without the snacks, there's a greater risk of low blood sugar.

If your child's current insulin therapy isn't designed according to the "basal/bolus" model, ask your doctor about it. There are times when it's not the best choice—for example, in infants who "graze" all day and don't eat meals or in youngsters who cannot take insulin injections during the school day. We talk about these sorts of situations throughout the book. But keep in mind that basal/bolus therapy is the gold standard of treatment for type 1 diabetes. It should be used whenever possible. By mimicking the body's normal insulin pattern, it improves our control and decreases the negative aspects of diabetes therapy. Basal/bolus insulin therapy also greatly simplifies diabetes nutrition, as you'll see later in this chapter.

Delivery Devices

Throughout the developed world, insulin pens are by far the most common delivery devices used by people with diabetes. They are more convenient and more accurate than syringes, but syringes are more common in the United States. Switching to a pen can reduce some of the burden and hassle associated with frequent injections. It may even help with control by improving the accuracy of dose delivery. If you're using syringes, talk to your doctor about the possibility of switching to a pen.

Another method of delivery is the insulin pump. Pumps are small beeper-sized devices that contain an insulin syringe. They pump insulin through the skin via a tiny tube and needle. The rate of insulin delivery is programmed into the pump, and the accuracy of the delivery is monitored mechanically. It's a great tool for basal/bolus therapy. Insulin pump use by kids has been growing dramatically in recent years because it can deliver very small amounts of insulin accurately and flexibly. But pumps are only as good as the brains running them, and extra training is needed to get their full benefit. If you are having ongoing challenges with basal/bolus therapy delivered by pen or syringe, you may want to discuss pump use with your doctor or team.

Changing How We Think about Diabetes and Food

All healthcare providers used to believe that someone with diabetes should control everything about their lives—especially food and exercise—to match prescribed insulin doses. Doses were seldom changed, and when they were, the doctor did it. This approach put good blood sugar control out of the reach of most people, since only the most consistently disciplined could manage it. It was difficult and the results were far from perfect. And things were even worse for people whose lives were *not* so regular or disciplined. In addition to poor control, they also struggled with stress and guilt over not being able to live such a structured life. Improvements in our treatment tools—better insulins, insulin delivery devices (pens and pumps), and home blood sugar monitoring tools—make it possible to match injected insulin to the situation. This change in thinking has not only made better control possible for more people but it has also reduced the amount of stress and restriction it takes to get there.

"One Size Fits All" Meal Plans Are No Longer Necessary

The new tools of insulin therapy make a new approach to food possible, too. Insulin regimens are now tailored to fit a person's usual eating habits. Both eating and insulin doses become dynamic—changing from day to day. In the more traditional approach, both insulin doses and food intake are kept constant, which requires following a specific meal plan. In Chapter 2, we described how such a plan can be developed, using a good record of what and when a child usually eats. We have included a lot of tools throughout the book for families who are still using this type of approach, but we encourage you to think of it as temporary. Moving toward a more flexible approach to food and insulin generally produces big rewards.

When the person with diabetes or his family learns how to count the carbohydrate in foods and to adjust insulin in response, insulin doses can change frequently, even with every meal. These timely insulin adjustments can greatly improve blood sugar control. They also give people greater flexibility—freedom to eat a wider variety of foods, to eat different amounts on different days, to sleep in occasionally, to do all sorts of spur-of-the-moment things—without losing blood sugar control.

Does this mean that your child can now forget about following a "diabetic diet"? That he can eat whatever he wants, whenever he wants? Yes and no. The child with diabetes needs the same healthy foods as everyone else. If he ate junk all the time, his health would suffer. This would still be true even if you and he could control his blood sugar while he did it. But since virtually any food can be included in a healthful eating plan, he *can* eat anything he wants, but not to the exclusion of other needed foods.

It will take some work. "Playing pancreas" is a demanding job. It means keeping track of what's eaten and then learning the specific effect of that food on blood sugar and insulin needs. How much insulin does it take to balance Grandma's chocolate birthday cake? Do they even make enough insulin to handle a large deep-dish pepperoni pizza? You can find the answers to these questions, just as you can deal with everyday meals. The process starts by understanding, in general, how different foods affect blood sugar.

The Effect of Foods on Blood Sugar and Insulin

All foods, except pure alcohol, add sugar to the blood, but not in equal amounts. Around 90 to 100 percent of digestible carbohydrates (starches and sugars) enters the bloodstream as glucose, but very little protein and fat are broken down into glucose. The glucose from carbohydrates tends to show up in the bloodstream shortly after eating, while glucose from proteins and fats tends to appear in the blood several hours later. Therefore, the amount of insulin needed to control blood sugar after meals depends mostly on the amount of carbs eaten. To understand diabetes nutrition and keep food and insulin in balance, you need to know how much carbohydrate your child eats.

Where's the Carbohydrate?

Carbohydrate is found in varying amounts in:

- Fruits and vegetables and the juices made from them
- Grain products, such as breads, rice, cereal, and pasta
- Starchy vegetables, such as potatoes, sweet potatoes, peas, and corn
- Dried or canned beans, peas, and lentils
- Dairy and soy products, particularly milk and yogurt (including soy milk)
- Sugar-sweetened foods, such as cake, candy, cookies, ice cream, and soda

Although all of these foods can be part of a healthful diet (*but in different proportions, as described in Chapter 3*), all foods add sugar to the bloodstream. They need to be balanced by insulin and/or exercise, or they will drive blood sugar far above the normal range. Not everyone manages this balancing act the same way.

Diabetes Meal-Planning Tools

The most common diabetes meal-planning tools are the carbohydrate counting and food exchange systems. They both work. So do less common systems, such as those that use calorie points or total available glucose (TAG), among others. Personally, we think that carbohydrate counting gives you and your child more flexibility in food choices and is a bit easier to learn than the other approaches. But you, your dietitian, or other healthcare provider may prefer some other system, which is also fine. In whatever system you use, you just need to know how all the foods your family eats are counted, so that insulin can be balanced with the carbohydrate content of what's eaten.

Food Exchange System

The Diabetes Food Pyramid, which we described earlier as a guideline for healthy eating, can be your bridge between family meals and diabetes meal planning. Look at the Diabetes Food Pyramid in Figure 4.1. It shows how the pyramid relates to food exchanges and carbohydrate counting. Notice how the sections of the pyramid correspond to the

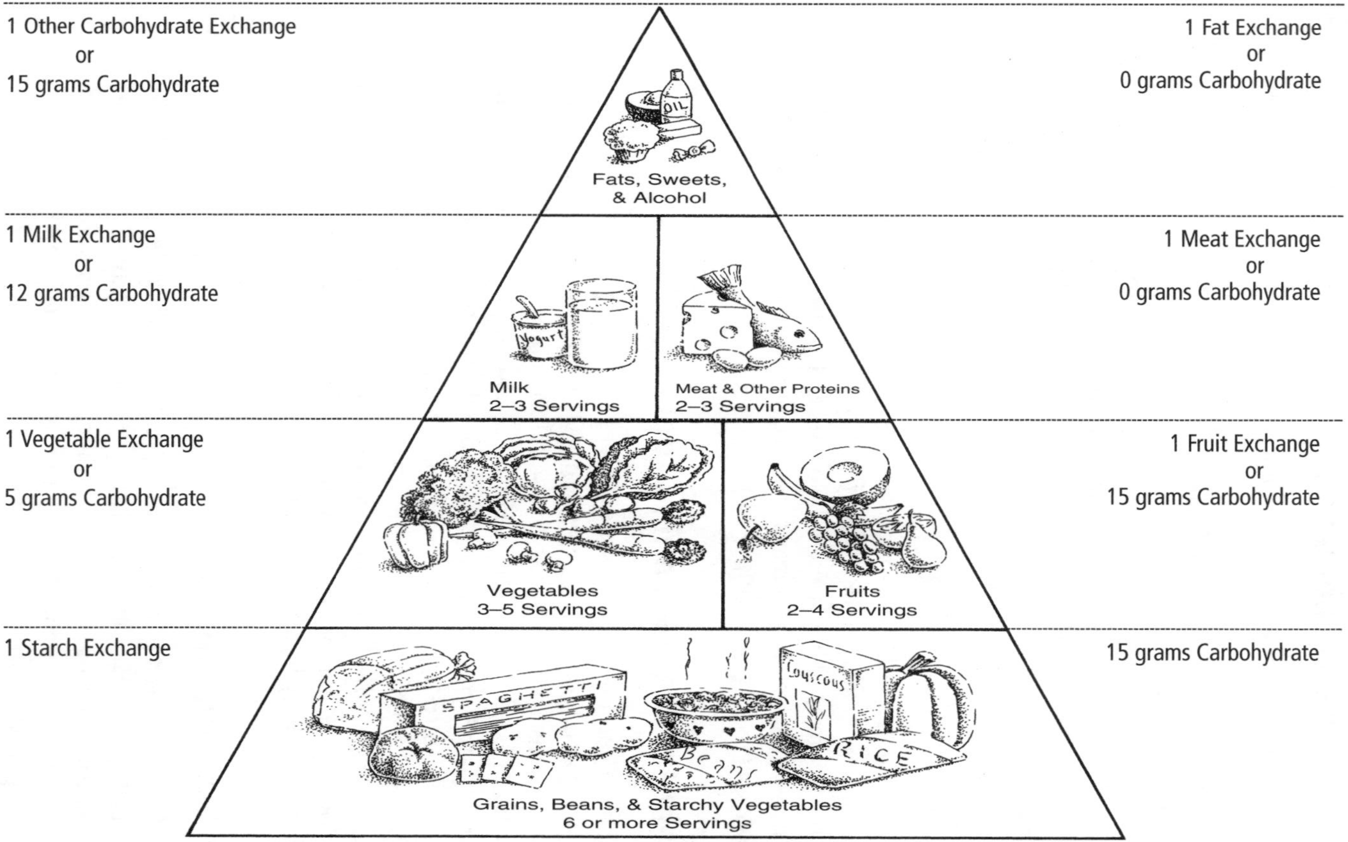
1 Other Carbohydrate Exchange
or
15 grams Carbohydrate
1 Fat Exchange
or
0 grams Carbohydrate
Fats, Sweets, & Alcohol
OIL
1 Milk Exchange
or
12 grams Carbohydrate
1 Meat Exchange
or
0 grams Carbohydrate
Yogurt
Milk
2–3 Servings
Meat & Other Proteins
2–3 Servings
1 Vegetable Exchange
or
5 grams Carbohydrate
1 Fruit Exchange
or
15 grams Carbohydrate
Vegetables
3–5 Servings
Fruits
2–4 Servings
1 Starch Exchange
15 grams Carbohydrate
SPAGHETTI
Couscous
Beans
RICE
Grains, Beans, & Starchy Vegetables
6 or more Servings

DIABETES FOOD PYRAMID

American Diabetes Association/The American Dietetic Association

FIGURE 4.1

food exchange groups and how a carbohydrate value can be assigned to servings from each pyramid group. If you use the Diabetes Food Pyramid to plan meals for the whole family, you can also use it to keep track of the carbohydrate your child is eating.

With food exchanges, the meal plan is made up of a given number of servings from each of three major food groups: carbohydrate, meat and meat substitutes, and fat. Table 4.1 shows how foods are divided into groups in the food exchange system and the average nutrient content of a serving from each group.

Because it describes everything eaten, an exchange meal plan covers both general nutrition needs and diabetes control in a single tool. In a move toward greater flexibility, the 1995 revised version of the exchange system (the one shown here) encourages people to exchange among *all* the carbohydrate-containing food groups. But even with this change, some people say they find the exchange system confusing. This may be because they didn't don't get enough instruction to use them effectively. After all, several meal-planning approaches not related to diabetes—including Weight Watchers and Deal-A-Meal—have used this versatile meal-planning tool. Still, it's clearly not for everyone.

Carbohydrate Counting

Carbohydrate counting simply means keeping track of how much carbohydrate is in each food eaten. This information is then used to determine the dose of insulin to cover the meal. Carbohydrate counting can also be used with a set meal plan and unchanging insulin

TABLE 4.1 Food Groups of the Exchange System

	Carbohydrate g	Protein g	Fat g	Calories
Carbohydrate Group				
Starch	15	3	1 or less	80
Fruit	15	0	0	60
Milk	12	8	0–8	90–150
Other Carbohydrates	15	varies	varies	varies
Vegetables	5	2	0	25
Meat and Meat Substitutes Group	0	7	0–8	35–100
Fat Group	0	0	5	45

doses. In that case, the meal plan consists of a target number of either servings or grams of carbohydrate for each meal and snack. "Servings" are 15-gram carbohydrate portions. Any combination of foods and serving sizes that provides the given amount of carbohydrate can be chosen. Food labels, exchange lists, food composition books, or a combination of these sources can provide the needed information.

Table 4.2 illustrates how a food record is viewed in terms of the Diabetes Food Pyramid, the food exchange system, and carbohydrate counting. The record shown is an average day for Jody, the four-year-old you met in Chapter 3. This was Jody's usual menu at the time.

Sources of Nutrition Information

No matter what food management approach you and your team choose, you'll need information about the nutrient content of the foods your family eats. You'll use that information either to fit foods into a meal plan or to match the meal-related insulin to what's eaten. Chances are, your team will provide you with some tools to get you started: a list of the carbohydrate content of certain foods or an exchange food list.

Just because a food isn't included in the literature that came from your dietitian, don't think it can't be part of your child's menu. The world has an abundance of different foods, and they can all be enjoyed if you have the necessary information. Your child can enjoy a varied diet and still maintain diabetes control.

One of the best sources of information is the Nutrition Facts label that appears on packaged food in the United States. The content of the label is dictated by federal regulations, and it should be quite accurate. Most packaged and processed foods have one, listing the amounts of calories, carbohydrate, protein, and fat in a given portion of the food, as well as other information. Figure 4.2 shows a sample Nutrition Facts label for a low-fat granola bar.

The information you'll need might include the calorie, carbohydrate, fat, and protein values. Depending on the meal-planning system you're using, you may need one, two, or even all of those values to figure out how the food fits. If you're counting grams of carbohydrate, you can take the total carbohydrate value right off the label. If you're counting carbohydrate exchanges or servings, divide the total carbohydrate value on the label by 15 to get the number of "carbs" provided by one serving. If you're

TABLE 4.2 Jody's Usual Menu, Shown in Different Systems

Jody's Food Record	Pyramid	Exchanges	Carb Counting
Breakfast			
1/2 cup Cheerios	1 Bread/Grain	1/2 Carb (Bread)	7 g
1/2 cup 2% milk	1/2 Milk/Dairy	1/2 Carb (Milk)	6 g
1/4 banana	1 Fruit	1/2 Carb (Fruit)	7 g
3 oz. orange juice	1 Fruit	1 Carb (Fruit)	12 g
			Meal Total = 32 g
Morning Snack			
1 slice white toast	1 Bread/Grain	1 Carb (Bread)	16 g
2 tbs. peanut butter	1 Meat/Protein	1 Meat/Substitute	0 g
1/2 cup 2% milk	1/2 Milk/Dairy	1/2 Carb (Milk)	6 g
			Meal Total = 22 g
Lunch			
1 oz. hamburger patty on	1 Meat/Protein	1 Meat/Substitute	0 g
1/2 hamburger bun	1 Bread/Grain	1 Carb (Bread)	15 g
6 carrot and celery sticks	1 Vegetable	1 Carb (Vegetable)	5 g
1/2 cup milk	1/2 Milk/Dairy	1/2 Carb (Milk)	6 g
1 oatmeal raisin cookie	1 Bread/Grain	1 Carb (Bread)	10 g
			Meal Total = 36 g
Afternoon Snack			
1 soft pretzel stick with	1 Bread/Grain	1/2 Carb (Bread)	6 g
1 oz. soft cheese	1 Meat/Protein	1 Meat/Substitute	0 g
1/2 cup apple juice	1 Fruit	1 Carb (Fruit)	15 g
			Meal Total = 21 g
Dinner			
2 oz. baked chicken	1 Meat/Protein	2 Meat/Substitute	0 g
1/2 cup cooked carrots	1 Vegetable	1 Carb (Vegetable)	8 g
1/3 cup mashed potatoes	1 Bread/Grain	1 Carb (Bread)	12 g
1/2 cup vanilla pudding with	1 Sweet/Fat	1 Carb (Other) + 1 Fat	17 g
1 pineapple ring	1 Fruit	1/2 Carb (Fruit)	7 g
1/2 cup 2% milk	1/2 Milk/Dairy	1/2 Carb (Milk)	6 g
			Meal Total = 50 g
Bedtime Snack			
1 oz. sliced chicken on	1 Meat/Protein	1 Meat/Substitute	0 g
1 slice white bread	1 Bread/Grain	1 Carb (Bread)	15 g
1/2 cup milk	1/2 Milk/Dairy	1/2 Carb (Milk)	6 g
			Meal Total = 21 g

Nutrition Facts

Serving Size 1 bar

Servings per Container 10

Amount per Serving

Calories 110   Calories from Fat 20

	% Daily Value
Total Fat 2g	3%
Saturated Fat 0.5g	3%
Cholesterol 0mg	0%
Sodium 100mg	4%
Total Carbohydrate 22g	7%
Dietary Fiber 1g	4%
Sugars 10g	
Protein 2g	

FIGURE 4.2

using one of the other meal-planning systems, ask your dietitian or other healthcare provider how to use the information on the label.

Regardless of which system you're using, be sure to check the serving size shown on the label against the amount your child actually eats: Is it more, less, or the same? If necessary, adjust the nutrient values to the portion actually eaten.

Reliable food composition information can also be found in brochures from most national restaurant and fast-food chains. If you need even more information after trying all these sources, consider investing in a good book on food composition. (*See the reading list at the end of this chapter.*)

Blood Sugar Monitoring: Your Tool of Discovery

Matching carbohydrate intake with insulin doses is a pretty straight-forward concept, but it can be a lot more challenging in actual practice. You need to respond to a constantly changing situation: Blood sugars, physical activity, and menus vary. And many other things—some that we still don't understand—subtly or radically change the diabetes control game. To keep up with the ever-changing show, you need timely information to guide your decisions. That's the real process of making diabetes management work, and it absolutely depends on regular blood glucose monitoring. No other source of information is as necessary or as powerful.

How much testing you'll do depends on blood sugar goals, insulin regimen, financial issues, and your child's cooperation, among other things. Your diabetes team can help you work out the best plan. Most kids require a minimum of four tests (before meals and at bedtime) to achieve control throughout the day. Occasionally tests are done around 3 A.M. to check for overnight lows, and more tests are needed during illness and exercise. Some teams also recommend after-meal tests to check the match in doses and timing between food and insulin, which we think is particularly valuable. Was two units the right dose for a piece of toast, an egg, and a glass of milk? The only way to know for sure is to test within a couple of hours after eating.

Make Monitoring Pay

Regardless of how many tests you do, make sure you're getting the most from each one. First of all, record every number. You or your child can write them down, or you may rely on meter memory. But being able to compare them with each other and with insulin doses and food intake is absolutely vital. At first, you'll probably be looking at the numbers with your dietitian, nurse, doctor, or other team member, but eventually you'll need to learn how to interpret them on your own.

You'll be looking for patterns and relationships: patterns that are related to certain days of the week, times of day, or activities, as well as relationships among food, insulin dose, activity, and the resulting blood sugar. You'll probably start simply, perhaps following a written plan for adjusting insulin doses according to how much carbohydrate is eaten. But with a lot of practice, you will progress to taking multiple factors into account—not only food, but also current blood glucose, activity that came before, activity that will come after, and so on.

To get the maximum benefit from blood sugar testing, you also need to be clear about what the goals are for various times of the day and what to do about specific values. For example, a blood glucose of

100 mg/dl (5.5 mmol) is probably within your target range for a before-meal reading: No action is needed other than, maybe, breathing a sigh of relief! But the same reading at bedtime may be lower than what your team has determined is safe to go to bed on. You'll need to know what to do at times like these. (*Options for bedtime snacks are discussed in Chapter 6.*)

Unless you learn how to use and respond to the numbers, testing can be extremely frustrating. You'll need to know what to do about the results, which is one of the many reasons why it's so important to keep working with your team. They should teach you in a step-by-step fashion, just as you will ultimately teach these skills to your child.

But first, let's examine the match between your child's eating and his insulin doses.

Adjusting Insulin to a Basic Meal Plan

Eventually, you will want to learn how to adjust insulin to changes in diet, but most people start out by learning a simpler method. The first step is to keep insulin doses the same each day and to balance food eaten with that set amount. With this method, you need to follow a specific meal pattern or plan. Consistently eating the same amount of carbohydrate at each meal and snack makes it much easier to fine-tune insulin doses and timing because there are fewer variables to consider when you review blood sugars. In general, the more the meal plans vary during this learning period, the longer it will take to figure out the right doses for both background and meal-related insulin. You might stick with this approach for just a few weeks or continue it for a longer period, depending on your situation and the recommendations of your healthcare team.

But consistency is not always easy to come by. Children's appetites vary from day to day. And clearly, food should not be forced or withheld when the child's appetite is out of sync with the meal plan. However, if the child is old enough to understand and cooperate, some simple adjustments can make it easier to keep carbohydrate intake stable, despite variations in appetite. These techniques can take some of the sting out of a set meal plan during the stage when insulin and food relationships are being worked out and families are not yet ready to start adjusting insulin on their own.

Sticking to a Meal Plan When Appetite Varies

When a child is still hungry after eating the food on the meal plan, foods with little or no carbohydrate can be added without affecting blood sugar levels. Try foods like celery and other raw vegetables, diet gelatin, meat, cheese, peanuts, and seeds. For example, if Jody was still hungry at lunchtime after eating her usual half a sandwich, vegetable sticks, milk, and cookie (*see Table 4.2*), her mom could let her choose peanut butter on celery sticks, a slice of cheese, or a handful of peanuts. None of these foods is likely to raise Jody's blood sugar very much, but they would taste good and satisfy her hunger.

On the other hand, if Jody wasn't hungry and couldn't finish the usual meal, her mom could give priority to the carbohydrates, perhaps removing some meat or vegetables from the table when she saw that Jody wasn't as hungry as usual. Or she could give the carbohydrates in a more concentrated form. She could substitute fruit juice for the milk—giving the same amount of carbohydrate in a smaller volume.

Choices Can Help Promote Consistency

Helping your child eat the planned amount of food (whether measured in grams or servings of carbohydrate, number of exchanges, or calorie points) is a key part of daily diabetes management if you're working with set insulin doses. This is less of an issue if you are adjusting rapid-acting insulin (Humalog or Novolog) for mealtimes. The decision about how much to eat will have already been made, and the child usually won't change his mind in the middle of the meal. (Of course, kids can and do change their minds midstream, but it is less likely to happen during a meal than when 30–45 minutes have elapsed between the insulin and the food.) If you are trying to follow a meal plan to which your child's set insulin dose is matched, the struggle comes up more often. The child either hates what you're having for dinner or wants to eat the whole casserole because he loves it so much. Given what we've said about the problems associated with either forcing or withholding food, what's the answer?

Parents tell us that choice makes all the difference. By offering a variety of choices that are all acceptable, you can get away from the "eat it or else" threat. Instead of having only one carbohydrate choice on the table, routinely offer two or three and make at least one of them something you're sure your kid will eat. Milk, applesauce, canned peaches, white bread, instant mashed potatoes, creamed corn, and fruit yogurt are stand-bys for younger children, and older kids may have their own preferences. When a child is given choices instead of ultimatums, he's a lot less likely to refuse to eat.

In addition, always offer some choices that don't raise blood sugar much, so your child can have more to eat if she's still hungry. Second helpings of the meat or other protein, vegetables with dip, green salad, nuts, and other low-carbohydrate foods are some options. Large amounts of fat or protein may raise blood sugar some hours afterward, however. Fats slow down the digestion of carbohydrates, and a small portion of protein can be converted to glucose under certain circumstances. Generally, though, these foods have far less effect on blood sugar than carbohydrate does.

If you are working with set insulin doses and a corresponding meal plan but your child frequently wants much more or less food than is planned, don't keep struggling. Talk to your dietitian or other diabetes educator about learning to adjust either the insulin for variable food intake or the current meal plan so it's a better fit.

How Do Sweets Fit Into Diabetes Management?

The carbohydrate in sweets certainly needs to be counted, whether you're fitting it into a set meal plan or using the count to calculate an insulin dose. Both the exchange and carbohydrate-counting systems make it easy to do this. We think one of the best ways to handle sweets is to put out the dessert at the beginning of the meal with everything else. Just set the dessert plate near the dinner plate. Will kids eat dessert first if you do this? Maybe. But if the serving size is appropriate, the child will still be hungry after polishing off a small piece of cake and will then eat the rest of the meal. And if you do this consistently, the novelty will eventually wear off.

We like this method because it avoids making sweets into something so special that you have to eat all the healthier foods to get them. It's as valuable for the other kids in the family as it is for the one with diabetes. Sweets become just another part of a healthy diet—something we enjoy in modest amounts without guilt. In terms of diabetes management, it conveys clearly that all carbohydrate foods are equally important to diabetes control. For this to work best, make sure that the amount makes sense for the child's age and appetite, so you don't displace nutritious foods from your child's diet.

How Important Are Portion Sizes?

Portion sizes are key. After all, knowing how much carbohydrate is eaten enables us to keep insulin matched to needs. Anyone who is playing pancreas needs that information. How precise you need to be, however, varies. Generally, the smaller the body size, the more important it is to be precise. A given amount of carbohydrate—say, 15 grams—will raise blood sugar a lot more in a 40-pound body than it will in a 120-pound body. But body weight is not the only factor. Kids of the same weight can respond differently to the same amount of carbohydrate, just as they might have quite different total insulin doses. Experience will show you what you need to do.

You may end up counting every gram of carbohydrate, roughly estimating exchange-size servings, or taking some middle ground. Whatever approach works for you, we hope that managing or counting portions will not be tied to *limiting* what your child eats. The purpose of paying attention to portions is to know how much carbohydrate he takes in so you can keep food and insulin in sync. Can you accomplish this without being the old ogre that counts out exactly 11 Teddy Grahams to a hungry child? We think so.

Easier Portion Management

One way to manage portion sizes is to fill everyone's plates before bringing them to the table, restaurant style. Another is to establish portions before cooking, by making individual casseroles, for instance. You can also serve foods in dishes that help you control serving size—for example, always filling the cereal or the fruit bowl to the same level or finding a small plate or bowl that holds your child's standard portion. What if the amount that your child wants to eat isn't the same as the serving size for which you have information? Figure it out. Say the little dessert plate actually holds 16 or 17 Teddy Grahams. (Pour a portion out two or three times, count or measure each one, and then take the average.) Use simple multiples or fractions of the value you know. If

11 Teddy Grahams equals one starch exchange or 14 grams of carbo-hydrate, count your little dessert plate serving as 1 1/2 starches or 21 grams of carbohydrate.

Prepackaged portions can also be helpful. Try individually wrapped granola bars (instead of a whole plate full of cookies), single cups of yogurt, or ice cream bars (instead of serving out of a gallon container). Those prepackaged portions are nearly always labeled, so you know exactly how much carbohydrate they contain.

Serving spoons that dish out a known amount are another helpful tool. For older kids, a serving spoon that holds half a cup might be useful because so many carbohydrate foods have a standard serving size of 1/2 cup. That same half-cup serving spoon can also be used to estimate other sizes of servings (a scant spoonful is 1/3 cup, half a spoonful is 1/4 cup, two spoonfuls is a cup, and so on). For toddlers and preschoolers, it may make more sense to use a tablespoon, rather than a serving spoon, as your standard measure. Half-cup portions can be overwhelming for little guys.

Simple techniques like these can help you keep servings consistent. If the portion sizes are the same, even if they're not measured exactly, you'll get the insulin adjusted to the serving size over time. The portion sizes become a habit that kids pick up.

Some people weigh and measure portions until they become familiar with portion sizes. However, many people who have done this tell us that portions eventually tend to grow until they are nowhere near the intended size. Therefore, those who estimate portions by eye should occasionally go back to measuring. Some families find it easier to just continue weighing and measuring.

A useful trick for kids and adults alike is to use their fist as a refer-ence. Most adult fists are about the volume of a cup. Obviously, the corresponding measure for a child varies with their age and size. But it can still be helpful because, as the man who taught us this says, "You always have your hands with you, and they're always the same size!" At home, have youngsters compare known portions to their fist. Then, when they're away from home, they can compare servings to their fist to try to get approximately the same amount that they already know the insulin dose or carbohydrate count for. It's a lot less hassle than carrying measuring cups around with you.

The families that are most successful seem to be the ones who find ways to integrate portion control into their food serving and preparation routines. But whether you use these ideas or not, try to find methods that fit your family and lifestyle.

Some Finer Points of Control

Timing Meals and Insulin

Blood sugar control is best when insulin is matched in both amount and timing with the glucose, or sugar, from digested food. Optimal timing depends on the type of insulin being used to cover the meal. For example, if regular insulin is taken too close to a meal, the blood sugar level can rise too high right after the meal and fall too low later. Or, if your child is a slow eater, his blood sugar may fall too low while he's eating because the rapid-acting insulin (Humalog or Novolog) reached the bloodstream before enough carbohydrate had been eaten to balance its effect. Timing is as important as dose to good control.

Rapid-acting insulins. The easiest way to minimize the timing issue is to use a rapid-acting insulin for meals. As we've said, these insulins act much more like the body's own insulin than do any of the slower insulins. They peak 60 to 90 minutes after they're injected. If they're taken within a few minutes before or after a meal, they arrive in the blood right on schedule.

The slower insulins and meal timing. Timing is not as easy with regular or other longer-acting insulins. Traditionally, a child had to wait a given length of time following the injection before being allowed to eat, usually 30 to 45 minutes for regular (R), NPH (N), or Lente (L) insulin. The best timing for these insulins can only be worked out by studying an individual's blood sugar results after they've eaten. For example, if blood sugars are too high right after a meal but come down into the target range before the next meal, we know the dose is correct, but the timing could be better. One solution would be to wait longer between the shot and the meal. But most families can't stand to watch the clock while a hungry five-year-old whines. Luckily, there is another strategy that can work pretty well.

Food tricks to help with insulin timing. We already know that different foods affect blood sugar differently, and this can help us improve the match between a sluggish insulin and food. Carbohydrates tend to raise blood sugar fairly quickly, creating an immediate need for insulin. Protein and fat have a much slower and weaker effect on blood sugar. And foods with few or no calories don't raise blood sugar at all. We can delay insulin demand (when regular, NPH, or Lente insulins are taken close to the meal) by eating the carbohydrate foods at the end of the meal. Start with salad. Then serve the meat and vegetables. Leave the bread, potato, fruit, and other high-carbohydrate foods until last. Dividing the food up in this way makes the biggest need for insulin hit closer to when regular and other longer-lasting insulins are peaking.

What about the child who eats slowly, or when insulin is taken and then dinner is delayed for some reason? In the first case, a rapid-acting insulin could be given after the pokey eater is done. And delayed meals are not a problem of rapid-acting insulin—provided the background insulin dose is correct—because it's not usually given until you actually sit down to eat. But these situations are a little trickier for those using regular insulin. When you're worried about lows, the carbohydrate foods could be offered first and meat, salad, and vegetables last.

Insulin timing for different eating styles. Intervals between insulin and meals can be adjusted to fit a kid's eating style in other ways too. For fast eaters, a longer delay between regular insulin and the meal may work best, or try putting the carbohydrate foods at the end of the meal. A short interval may be best for a child whose appetite is poor or who eats slowly. In this situation, regular insulin could be given very close to the meal or even afterward. Neither of these is a perfect solution, but they can help keep the child's safe while keeping the family sane.

In such cases, you may want to have a long talk with your team about rapid-acting insulin for meal coverage. Be aware, however, that it won't be a solution for every child. Regular insulin may be a good choice for younger kids who still need to eat frequently (*see Chapter 6*). And some kids can't take an injection at school to cover lunch with rapid-acting insulin. But in our experience, rapid-acting insulin can help solve some common problems: reducing lows between meals and overnight, solving the insulin timing issue, and even making it possible to inject *after* meals, thus eliminating battles about how much food must be eaten.

Adjusting Insulin Doses for Eating

There is a relationship between the grams of carbohydrate your child eats and the amount of insulin his body needs to handle it. That ratio can be used to calculate the appropriate bolus (premeal dose of rapid-acting or regular insulin) for any meal or snack. The carbohydrate-to-insulin ratio varies quite a bit from person to person. Most children need about one unit of rapid-acting insulin for every 15 to 20 grams of carbohydrate. In general, the lower the total daily insulin dose, the greater the amount of carbohydrate covered by one unit of insulin. To find your child's unique value, start with an estimate and test it. Some people start with one unit for every 15 grams of carbohydrate, since this is the value of a carbohydrate exchange serving.

1. Test your child's blood sugar before eating. It should be in his target range. If it's too high or low, the effect of the insulin dose (premeal bolus) being tested will be unclear.

2. Count the carbohydrate that's being eaten. Use any meal that you know the total carbohydrate value for, such as 1 ounce of cereal, 8 ounces of milk, and 4 ounces of juice (which equals three carbohydrate portions, or 45 grams of carbohydrate).

3. Calculate the bolus for the meal using your estimated ratio. For example, 10-year-old Guy plans to eat the 45-gram carbohydrate meal described above. He's using an estimated ratio of one unit for every 15 grams of carbohydrate, so he'll take three units of rapid-acting insulin.

4. Test blood sugar after the meal and adjust the ratio as needed. The test can be done from one to three hours after the meal for rapid-acting insulin or from two to five hours after the meal for regular. If, for example, you want to keep your child's two-hour after-meal blood sugar values below 160 mg/dl (9 mmol), you might want to do the test two hours after the meal. Or if your goal is to have your child's blood sugars between 80 and 120 mg/dl (4–7 mmol) before meals, you might choose to just test before the next meal. If the reading is higher than the target value, then try a lower carbohydrate-to-insulin ratio (more insulin per amount of carbohydrate) at the next meal. For example, if Guy consistently had a two-hour postmeal blood glucose of more than 200 mg/dl (11 mmol) with the three-unit bolus, he might try using one unit of insulin for each 10 or 12 grams (instead of 15). On the other hand, if his blood sugar after eating was below the target range or he had low blood sugar, he would need to adjust the ratio so that he was getting *less* insulin for the same amount of carbohydrate. He could next try taking one unit for every 17 or 20 grams. He would continue testing and adjusting until he was reaching his glucose targets most of the time. (No one reaches his targets all the time!)

Once you and your child have figured out this relationship, you can calculate the correct insulin dose for any meal. You will be able to adjust for when your child is very hungry, when special occasions come along, or when he doesn't feel very hungry at all. Now *that's* flexibility!

Insulin and Food Adjustments for Out-of-Range Blood Sugars

Modifying mealtime insulin doses according to what's being eaten works best when the blood sugar at the beginning of the meal is in your child's target range. But that's not always the case. Blood sugar is often higher or lower than it's supposed to be. This happens because so many factors affect blood sugar and our treatment tools aren't perfect. To get the best possible blood sugar control, it's necessary to respond to those out-of-range readings when they happen.

One of the best tools for responding to out-of-range blood sugars is a specific plan (sometimes called an algorithm or sliding scale) for adjusting insulin based on the current blood sugar level. High blood sugar means there's too little insulin. So, in addition to whatever insulin will be taken to cover the meal, extra insulin is needed to correct the high blood sugar. Low blood sugar means there is already too much insulin, so less insulin can be given to cover the coming meal.

Some people "guesstimate" what those adjustments should be, giving one to two units more or less than the usual dose. Other folks don't make any adjustments at all. They may not know how, or they may have had a bad experience with it in the past. We feel that these adjustments are appropriate for most children with diabetes, but you need a rational and consistent approach. Your doctor or educator may have helped you determine the adjustment factor for your child, but if not, we have a simple way to identify one that should be fairly accurate.

A Step beyond Guessing

Years ago, Dr. Paul Davidson, an endocrinologist from Atlanta, found that people using regular insulin could estimate how much a single unit would decrease their blood sugar by using a mathematical constant of 1,500. Davidson's "1,500 Rule" says to divide the number 1,500 by the total daily insulin dose, which is the sum of *all* insulin taken in a 24-hour period. (Use 83 instead of 1,500 if you use mmol to measure blood sugar.)

Now that rapid-acting insulin is in wide use, some diabetes centers have modified this formula. They recommend using 1,800 (100 in the mmol system) as the constant for rapid-acting insulin because of its more concentrated effect. Rapid-acting insulin peaks much faster than regular and so lowers glucose faster.

For example, the total of all of 12-year-old Andy's insulin doses (all the rapid-acting meal insulin plus all the NPH) is 30 units. According to the "1,800 Rule," we would expect one unit of rapid-acting insulin to reduce Andy's blood sugar by about 60 mg/dl (3.3 mmol). Andy and his parents use that value to tweak his insulin doses before meals when his blood sugar is out of target range.

Let's say his blood sugar before supper is 288 mg/dl (16 mmol), but his target range is between 90 and 120 mg/dl (5–7 mmol) before meals. He'll need some extra insulin to correct that high blood sugar. Using his adjustment factor of one unit of rapid-acting insulin for every 60 mg/dl (3.3 mmol) of blood sugar, his parents calculate that he should add three units to his premeal dose. The extra three units should bring his blood sugar back to about 108 mg/dl (6.2 mmol). That would allow the meal-related insulin dose to really do its job. Without this adjustment, his blood sugar after the meal is likely to be just as high as or higher than it was before.

If Andy was on a set meal plan with a set meal bolus and couldn't finish his dinner (some children have reduced appetites when their blood sugar is high), there would be less need to increase the dose. (*See Table 4.3 for another example of how to calculate an insulin adjustment when blood glucose is above the target range.*)

TABLE 4.3 Calculating the Insulin Adjustment Factor for High Blood Sugar Using the 1,500 Rule for Regular Insulin

Lisa is eight years old. She takes 17 units of insulin a day (6 units of NPH [N] and 4 units of regular [R] before breakfast, 3 units of R before dinner, and 4 units of N at bedtime).

Calculating Lisa's Insulin Adjustment Factor:

1,500 ÷ 17 = 88 mg/dl (expected drop in blood glucose for each unit of R insulin). (In mmol system: 83 ÷ 17 = 4.9 mmol/unit of R)

Situation: Lisa's blood glucose
before supper is   252 mg/dl (14 mmol)
     − 120 mg/dl (6.7 mmol) (her highest blood glucose target
         before meals)
     = 132 mg/dl (difference ÷ 88 = 1 1/2 units of R insulin
         adjustment) OR
     7.3 mmol (difference ÷ 4.9 mmol = 1 1/2 units of R)

Solution: Add 1 1/2 units of R to Lisa's three-unit presupper dose to correct the high blood glucose.
     Adjusted dose = 4 1/2 units of R before supper

The same adjustment factor can also be used to reduce the premeal insulin dose if the blood sugar is too low before the meal. If Andy's blood sugar was only 60 mg/dl (3.3 mmol) before supper, his premeal dose based on the carbs to be eaten could be reduced by one unit to help correct the low. However, if Andy was extra hungry because of his low blood sugar, he might just want to eat more.

Some doctors want you to delay the meal until the premeal insulin has brought a very high blood sugar down closer to the target range. This works, but it can be really hard with a hungry child. You can get some of the same effect without having to wait to eat by following our earlier suggestion of first offering things that don't raise the blood sugar (salad, vegetables, meat). Leave the carbohydrate foods until the end of the meal, when the insulin has had some time to start working on that high blood sugar.

Making insulin and food adjustments is a skill that you and your child can develop through trial, error, and a lot of practice. Your doctor or educator may be a good resource to help you troubleshoot any difficulties that arise.

If You Don't Want to Adjust Insulin

If you're not yet comfortable making insulin adjustments, you can try modifying eating instead. This is not usually as satisfactory as making an insulin adjustment, but it can work if your child will cooperate. As you know, trying to keep a hungry child from eating, even when blood sugars are high, is likely to start a battle. You can try offering more low-carbohydrate foods and fewer high-carbohydrate ones to minimize the insulin demand. But keep in mind that kids may start withholding information about high sugars if parents routinely hold back food when blood sugars are high. On the other hand, they usually like getting the extra food when sugars are low.

Pattern-Based Insulin Adjustments

When you see a consistent pattern of high or low blood sugars over the course of two or three days, it makes sense to correct the pattern instead of constantly adjusting for it. Say Andy needed two or three extra units of insulin at dinnertime for three days in a row because of a high blood sugar. On the fourth day, a couple of units could be added to the basic dose of insulin responsible for the reading at that time of day. In his case, it would be his morning dose of NPH. For another child, it might be a prelunch dose of regular. This approach is sometimes called a pattern-based insulin adjustment.

Find a Way to Deal with Out-of-Range Sugars

Finding comfortable, workable ways to respond to daily blood sugar readings is key to better blood sugar control. After all the time, discomfort, and money you invest in blood sugar testing, it seems a waste just to gather up the numbers in a book for the doctor or nurse to review every few months—much of the power of those tests is lost when the information isn't used right away. There isn't much that the doctor can do about highs or lows when she sees the numbers weeks or months after the fact.

Recommended Reading and Resources

Food Pyramids

The First Step in Diabetes Meal Planning. American Diabetes Association/The American Dietetic Association, Alexandria, VA (1997).

The Food Guide Pyramid. United States Department of Agriculture, Human Nutrition Information Service, U.S. Government Printing Office, Washington, D.C. (2000).

Exchange Meal Planning

Exchange Lists for Meal Planning. American Diabetes Association/The American Dietetic Association, Alexandria, VA (1995).

Exchanges for All Occasions, by Marion Franz, RD, MS. International Diabetes Center, Minneapolis (2000).

Carbohydrate Counting

Carbohydrate Counting: A Primer for Insulin Pump Users to Zero In on Good Control, by Karmeen Kulkarni, Linda Fredrickson, and Marilyn Graff. Medtronics MiniMed, Sylmar, CA (2000).

Getting Started (introduces concepts), *Moving On* (introduces pattern reading), and *Using Carbohydrate/Insulin Ratios* (adjusting insulin for changes in food or activity). American Diabetes Association, Alexandria, VA (1995).

Complete Guide to Carbohydrate Counting, by Hope Warshaw and Karmeen Kulkarni. McGraw-Hill, New York (2001).

Food Composition

Bowes and Church's Food Values of Portions Commonly Used, by Jean A.T. Pennington, PhD, RD. 17th edition. Lippincott, Williams and Wilkins, Philadelphia (1998).

The Complete Book of Food Counts, by Corrinne Netzer. 4th edition. Fine Communications (1997).

Fast Food Facts, by Marion Franz. International Diabetes Center, Minneapolis (1997).

THE BOTTOM LINE

1. Food intake is inseparable from glucose control.
2. To ensure both blood sugar control and normal childhood growth, insulin doses should be matched to calorie needs, not the other way around.
3. If a meal plan is used, it should mirror the child's usual eating habits.
4. Carbohydrate—starches and sugars—are the main source of blood glucose.
5. Keep track of all carbohydrate so that insulin can be kept in balance with intake.
6. Offering lots of choices promotes consistency without turning Mom and Dad into the "food police."
7. To get the most flexibility and best control, learn to adjust insulin for changes in food eaten.
8. Learn to adjust insulin for out-of-range blood sugars using the 1,800 Rule; 1,500 Rule; or guidelines from your healthcare provider.

5

Beyond Blood Sugar Control: Diabetes Goals for Families

A t age 15, Nicole was having a hard time: with her diabetes, with her doctor, and with her very frustrated parents. The pursuit of perfect blood sugar control was at the center of the storm. An advocate of good control, Nicole's doctor had always examined her blood sugar records closely at every visit. She circled every number above 160 or below 70 mg/dl and then asked for an explanation of what had gone wrong. With a lot of hard work and dedication from both of Nicole's parents, this approach had consistently produced A1C values of less than eight percent ever since her diagnosis at the age of seven.

The A1C test, also known as the glycosylated hemoglobin or glycohemoglobin test, measures average blood sugar control over the past two to three months according to how much sugar clings to red blood cells. The higher the blood sugar, the more "candy coating" on the cells.

Unfortunately, things had started to change about the time that Nicole turned 13, and they had been getting steadily worse ever since.

When Mom or Dad forced her to do a blood test and the result was a high reading, it usually led to a fight.

75

The first sign of a problem had been more variability in her home blood sugar test readings—higher highs, lower lows, and more of both. Then her A1C numbers started to climb. This triggered a lot of questions from both the doctor and her parents. They accused Nicole of not following her meal plan or of not taking her insulin when she was away from home. Soon, she started "forgetting" to do her blood tests. When Mom or Dad forced her to do a blood test and the result was a high reading, it nearly always led to a fight. By the time we saw them, Nicole was meeting her parents' questions with stony silence.

"She doesn't follow a meal plan at all anymore," her father said. "She has an after-school job, and I think she spends most of the money she makes eating at fast-food places with her friends. I keep telling her she's going to get complications, but she doesn't care. She just wants to do things with her friends. We're worrying about her diabetes all the time now, because she never does."

Her parents' worry and frustration were understandable—they just wanted her to be healthy. But what does *healthy* really mean when your child has diabetes? It means good blood sugar control, of course. But it means much more than that, too. It means being happy and self-confident, at least most of the time. It means that your child cares about things, and that she works hard at the things she cares about. That's the ideal; the reality is often dramatically less glowing. All too often, it seems like the blood sugar part of your child's health is on a collision course with all the other parts, and that a big pile-up is always just ahead. This is a problem every parent of a child with diabetes faces constantly. Isn't there some way out of this fix? Isn't there a way to help your child be healthy in every way? It might be hard to believe, but the answer is yes.

How Important Is Good Blood Sugar Control?

Immediate benefits. Keeping blood sugars as close to normal as possible is extremely important. For one thing, it has immediate benefits. Most children feel awful when their blood sugars are bouncing around. Low blood sugar (hypoglycemia) is always uncomfortable and sometimes embarrassing, scary, or even dangerous. Some children also feel rotten when their blood sugar is too high (hyperglycemia), but children are less likely than adults to say they feel bad at these levels. Adults often feel exhausted and cranky when their sugar levels are high, while many kids say they feel fine or even have more energy. If your child feels fine when her sugar levels are high, it may be hard to convince her that high blood sugars can hurt her. Most kids live and think very much in the present moment. Those long-term complications you worry about all the time don't impress them as much.

When your child's blood sugars are low she probably feels bad, and it's hard for her to function. When the brain runs out of glucose—the only fuel it can use—it can't work well. It starts to sputter and stall like a car running out of gas. She may have trouble concentrating and relating to other people and may become uncoordinated. If her blood sugar gets really low, she may even pass out.

Recent studies show that high blood sugars can affect how your child functions as well. When people get hyperglycemic, they do things more slowly and make more mistakes.

Long-term benefits. The long-term benefits of good blood sugar control are undeniable. The body needs plenty of energy and the right amount of insulin to grow, and good control is key to normal growth and development in children.

The Diabetes Control and Complications Trial

We now know that good control is essential for minimizing the risk of long-term complications. In 1993, the results of the 10-year Diabetes Control and Complications Trial (DCCT) were released. This study was designed to answer two vital questions. First, if people treated their diabetes intensively, would their blood sugar control improve? Second, if their control improved, would they lower their risk of developing diabetes-related complications?

To answer these questions, people between the ages of 13 and 39 with type 1 diabetes were recruited from all over the United States and Canada. Half of them were assigned to the intensive treatment group. They took at least three shots a day or used an insulin pump, and they tested their blood sugar at least four times a day. They also spoke and met as often as they needed to with diabetes educators—primarily nurses and dietitians. The educators provided whatever training, advice, and support people needed to actively manage their own daily care. As a result of this emphasis on self-management, most people in this group learned to adjust their own insulin doses to get the best possible control between medical visits. Their goal was to get their blood sugar as close to normal as they could without causing too much low blood sugar.

The remaining DCCT participants received what was at that time conventional or typical treatment for people with type 1 diabetes. People in the conventional treatment group took one or two insulin shots a day, did some blood sugar testing, and saw the doctor every three months. Their goal was to control their diabetes well enough to be free of symptoms and to grow properly.

Is better control possible? We can still remember sitting in a throng of 5,000 at the American Diabetes Association's annual meeting when the final results were discussed. It was a thrilling moment. First, we learned that people in the intensive treatment group did achieve better blood sugar control. The upper limit of normal on the A1C test used in the study was 6.05 percent. In the first six months of the study, the average A1C of the intensive treatment group dropped from 9.0 percent (an average blood sugar of about 230 mg/dl) to 7.2 percent (an average blood sugar of about 155 mg/dl). It stayed at that lower level throughout the 10 years of the study. Adolescents in the study had slightly higher A1C levels than adult participants in both groups; however, their results showed comparable improvements. In the conventional treatment group, blood sugar stayed about where it had started (A1C was 9.0 percent and average blood sugar was about 230 mg/dl). Researchers could thus conclude that if people treated their diabetes intensively, their blood sugar control would improve.

Does this improved control prevent complications? We were not surprised to find that better blood sugar control meant fewer complications. Smaller studies and our own experience had already convinced most of us. What did surprise us, however, was how big a difference intensive treatment made. In the DCCT, intensive treatment reduced eye disease by as much as 76 percent. It also reduced kidney disease, decreasing the development of early kidney problems by 35 percent and more advanced kidney problems by 56 percent. Nerve damage was reduced by 60 percent.

Do these results apply to kids? The DCCT has proven that good blood sugar control is possible and that this control will help prevent complications in relatively young adults with type 1 diabetes—the type of people who were in the DCCT. However, no children younger than 13 participated in the study, and there were only 190 teenagers, so the DCCT doesn't tell us exactly what we should be doing about control in young kids. Even so, using a little common sense and what we know about development, we can figure it out. We think tight blood sugar control should be a priority for your child, as long as you realize that it will never be perfect and that there are certain risks.

What's Realistic for Children and Blood Sugar Control?

The goal for DCCT's intensive treatment group was normal blood sugar control, and every effort was made to help people achieve this goal. But despite this, only 20 percent of the intensive treatment group ever had a normal glycohemoglobin reading during the entire study, and only 5 percent had normal values throughout the study. Clearly, most people who have diabetes just can't achieve totally normal blood sugars. In addition, among the teenagers in the DCCT intensive treatment group, the proportion who achieved normal glycohemoglobin readings was even lower than among adults. As the parent of a child with diabetes, this probably comes as no surprise to you.

Don't expect perfection. All this suggests that perfection, or completely normal blood sugar values, is not a realistic goal when you have diabetes. And it's especially unrealistic when the person with diabetes is a child.

Years ago, a man named Lawrence Pray, who had been diagnosed with diabetes in the 1940s at the age of seven, wrote a book entitled *Journey of a Diabetic*. In his book, Pray offered some wise counsel: "Don't try for perfection. Try for good control, to be sure, but perfection lasts a moment, and diabetes lasts a lifetime." Perfection is impossible. If you try to achieve it, you won't succeed, and it will only make you (and your child) frustrated and miserable. This is especially true for children with diabetes, because their blood sugar levels often fluctuate even more dramatically than the levels of adults. And among all children, teenagers often have the hardest time with blood sugar control.

We used to think these difficulties arose because teenagers "act out" more than younger children or adults. Now we know that this is only part of the story. All those raging hormones of adolescence also play their part in teenage blood sugar instability. Growth hormones and stress hormones, which flow in abundance during adolescence, counteract the effects of insulin, pushing blood sugar levels up and making control harder to achieve.

"Good enough" control. It's important to set realistic, as well as ambitious, goals for your child's blood sugar control. Go for control that is "good enough," rather than perfect. Remember that the people in the DCCT who did well still had A1C levels of about 7 percent, which was a full percentage point above the normal range and equals an average blood sugar of about 155 mg/dl. Not perfect, but good enough. This "good enough" control (endorsed by the American Diabetes Association) will allow your child to feel well, grow and develop normally, and have less risk for complications.

It turns out that the relationship between blood sugar and the risk of complications among DCCT participants was pretty straightforward: The lower the blood sugar level, the lower the risk of complications, at every blood sugar level. This means that *any* improvement in your child's blood sugar control will probably lead to a reduced risk of complications. You don't need to reach some specific blood glucose value before you see a benefit. For example, if your child's A1C goes from 10 to 9 percent, her risk of complications drops about 30 percent. And it drops another 30 percent when her A1C goes from 9 percent to 8 percent. People who maintain A1C levels of 7 percent still have some chance of developing complications, but that risk is fairly low. Keeping levels below 7 percent is very difficult, especially for young people.

Risks of Better Glucose Control

Every benefit in life has a cost, and the risks of attempting better control include having more frequent low blood sugars, gaining weight, and letting diabetes dominate family life. You can minimize the risks, but you need to weigh them against the benefits before deciding to pursue better control.

More Frequent Low Blood Sugars

Skating close to the edge. People in the intensive treatment group of the DCCT had three times as much hypoglycemia as those in the standard treatment group. That should come as no surprise: When your goal is normal blood sugars, you don't have much margin for error. Think of a child walking around a deep lake. She is far more likely to fall in if she walks at the edge of the water than if she takes a path farther from the shore. In the same way, if your child's blood sugar is 140 mg/dl and it drops 80 points, to 60 (or if it is 7.8 mmol and drops 4.5, to 3.3 mmol), she is dangerously close to a low reaction. If her blood sugar drops the same 80 mg/dl (4.4 mmol) from a reading of 240 mg/dl (13.3 mmol), the result is a blood sugar of 160 (8.9 mmol), nowhere near the low range. The closer to normal it usually is, the more difficult it is to prevent low blood sugars: There is less room for error and for the sometimes surprising shifts in blood sugar caused by factors we don't understand or can't control.

Studies conducted since the DCCT confirm that kids with lower A1C levels tend to have more lows. Keep in mind, though, that the DCCT study was conducted using regular insulin for mealtimes—rapid-acting insulin had not been developed yet. In the years since Humalog and Novolog have become available, studies in adults have shown significantly less hypoglycemia at *all* A1C levels with these rapid-acting insulins, as compared to regular insulin. However, even if the risk is less with these newer insulins, people with near-normal blood sugars still run a greater risk of lows than if they would if they were keeping their blood sugars higher at all times.

Special risks for younger children. Hypoglycemia (which we discuss more fully in Chapter 7) is a special problem for children. For one thing, young children may have trouble recognizing when they are low and communicating what's going on. In addition, severe hypoglycemia, especially if it is frequent, can affect the developing brains of children under the age of seven or so. When a person is hypoglycemic, her brain is starved for fuel. In these very young children, the fuel is needed not just for immediate functioning but for brain development as well. But the effects are probably restricted to young children and the impact is hard to measure with any accuracy. Still, this concern reinforces the importance of not pushing for the lowest possible blood sugar levels.

Unwanted Weight Gain

Calories Aren't Voided. The second potential drawback of tight control—weight gain—was also documented in the DCCT. Those in the intensive treatment group gained an average of 10 pounds more over the course of the study than those in the conventional treatment group did. There are several possible reasons for this. One has to do with the blood sugar level itself. When blood sugar is high (above about 180 mg/dl or 10 mmol for most people), sugar ends up in the urine. Sugar in the urine contains calories that the body never had a chance to use, which is why weight loss is often a sign that diabetes control needs improvement. When control improves, the body hangs on to all the calories eaten, just as it does in people who don't have diabetes, so people may gain weight unless eating is reduced or activity increased. (In Chapter 9, we talk about the way some young people—mostly young women—purposely take less insulin in order to keep their weight down.)

Keep in mind that gaining some weight is normal when blood sugar control improves. The body can rehydrate and replace the muscle and fat that had been burned for energy while control was not good. However, if weight gain continues, the healthcare team should check out the entire diabetes management plan, including insulin doses, meal plans, and the frequency of low blood sugars.

More snacks to treat lows. Episodes of low blood sugar are treated with food, and these extra calories can cause weight gain. This is another good reason for preventing low blood sugars in the first place.

Eating more freely. When people get really good at controlling blood sugars, they can make more-liberal food choices. They learn how to eat sweets and other favorite foods while still keeping blood sugars in control, but these high-calorie foods may cause weight gain, just as they might in someone without diabetes.

Does the Complications Clock Tick More Slowly during Childhood?

Our children with diabetes have so many years ahead to live with the disease that we worry about the unseen damage that could be done. However, some people believe that during the years before adolescence, the "complications clock" ticks more slowly than it does in later years; there is no clear evidence of this, but it may help you feel a little less pressured as you work out an effective plan for helping your child manage her diabetes.

Avoiding Disharmony and Finding Solutions for Your Family

Any workable plan for living with diabetes must take into account your family's unique strengths and vulnerabilities. You also need to consider your schedules, the personalities of family members, and the support you have for coping with day-to-day stresses. If you are a single working parent with several children to care for and no family or friends to lighten your load, your plan will be quite different than if you are a two-parent family with only one child and lots of support. (*See Chapters 13 and 14 for tips on keeping family members sane.*)

Balancing Control with Other Important Goals

Here's the way we see the overall goal: raising a normal (as much like other kids as possible), healthy, emotionally strong, independent child who will be able to deal with all the challenges life presents—those that come from diabetes and those that don't. As you know only too well, working toward that goal is a difficult balancing act.

Your family's goals. Each family must work out for itself what its goals and plans are, depending on its lifestyle, values, and resources. When you find your answer, diabetes will assume its proper place in your family's life: important but not all-consuming. For instance, sometimes the pursuit of tight blood sugar control becomes so strong that it starts to dominate family life. Finding the right balance is a continuing process for most families. They get there for a while and then something changes that puts the diabetes back in the driver's seat again. When that happens, they need to once again make adjustments so they are controlling the diabetes and not the other way around.

Good blood sugar control goes hand in hand with emotional health and independence. It's actually a package deal: You either get both or you get neither. To get both, you and your child must work together.

Helping Your Child Learn to Care for Herself

You may feel like you are responsible for controlling your child's blood sugars, but it's not true. Your real job, if you want your child to have a healthy, happy life, is to help her learn to control her own blood sugars.

When you take responsibility for solving all the problems involved in managing your child's diabetes, two things happen. First, you deprive her of the opportunity to learn how to solve her own problems. She will need that skill throughout her life, and it can only be developed through practice. Second, when you take full responsibility for controlling your child's diabetes, she is left with only one way to exert her own control—by resisting you. The result is usually a deadlock, with everyone miserable. The following story illustrates the approach we advocate.

Sally's story. Sally was six years old when she was diagnosed with diabetes, just a few weeks before the winter holiday season. Along with the many painful adjustments the family faced, there was the prospect of giving up some precious family traditions—like baking Christmas cookies. Sally's mom was convinced that baking the cookies would be courting disaster because Sally would gorge herself on them, as she had in the past. Sally's mom was taking responsibility for controlling her daughter's blood sugars. And who could blame her? But the result was that Sally felt deprived and resentful. Her mother felt guilty for denying her daughter and angry at the same time. The rest of the family just didn't know what to do.

Let's try an experiment. When Sally and her mom brought up this dilemma on a visit to Sally's diabetes clinic, the counselor suggested an experiment. Instead of Mom having to solve the problem for her, Sally should be given the responsibility. This seemed like a pretty radical idea to both of them, but they were willing to give it a try. The rules of the experiment were that Sally could suggest any solution to the problem and her mom could accept it, offer another one, or say no. Her mother had to promise not to put Sally down for her suggestions, no matter how outrageous they might seem. She had to say no matter-of-factly, in a way that encouraged Sally to come up with another suggestion. If Mom heard a suggestion that she agreed with in part but believed was not the whole answer, she could suggest a modification to Sally. Then Sally could either say yes, no, or offer her own counterproposal.

Possible solutions. Sally and her mom quickly got the hang of the experiment, the essence of which is working cooperatively to solve a family problem. After offering a few possible solutions that her mom turned down, Sally suggested that she be allowed to have one cookie a day during the holidays.

Her mother just couldn't believe Sally would accept her daily cookie and not whine for more. Sally, for her part, was certain that she could accept her limit, adding that one cookie a day was better than none.

From the mouths of babes. The counselor saw possibilities here and jumped in to ask Sally to suggest a consequence if she couldn't follow her agreement. Sally immediately said, "We could take all the rest of the cookies and give them to the neighbors." At this, her mom laughed and agreed to give it a try. When asked what the rest of the family would say if their Christmas cookies suddenly disappeared, Sally's mom smiled, saying, "I'll just make it clear to them from the start what the deal is. Either we'll all have cookies, or none of us will."

Do your job and help your child do hers. This approach works because you assume your proper responsibility and allow your child to do the same. It's your child's job to learn how to control her diabetes. And it's your job to help her learn and to protect her from hurting herself in the process. In our experience, this approach works, even with children as young as four or five.

Let's say your five-year-old son was looking forward to ice cream for dessert. You test his blood before dinner, and it's at 320 mg/dl. Your natural response is, "No ice cream tonight!" Then what happens? Your child gets upset, and you get upset, too. All too often the real issue, how to manage your child's food when his blood sugar level is high, gets lost in the ensuing uproar.

Even a five-year-old child can begin to solve these problems. You can remind him what the real problem is: It's not safe to let his blood sugars go any higher, and the ice cream might do that. Then you can ask him what he thinks the right approach might be. Think of the way Sally and her mother worked together. If your child suggests eating the ice cream anyway, you can tell him that won't work and encourage him to think of another idea. If he gets frustrated and says he can't think of anything or gets upset and says he just won't have any, you can tell him you're sorry he can't think of anything that would work. If you have any ideas yourself, you could offer them. (Remember, he can reject your ideas, just as you are free to reject his.)

A powerful lesson. When this approach is used consistently, kids quickly get the idea: They can have something they want if they can figure out how to do it safely. Your child might suggest extra insulin to correct the high blood sugar and cover the ice cream. Or he might suggest some exercise after dinner and before dessert. Or saving the ice cream for tomorrow. Whatever he suggests, you can accept, offer a counterproposal, or say no. If he offers a solution that appeals to you, a few extra units of rapid-acting insulin, for instance, you can even ask him how many units he suggests. If he says three units but you think two would be better, you can suggest he start with two (to protect him from going too low), and when you test his blood at bedtime you both can tell how good your guesses were. You can use this information the next time you face the same problem. Even more important, the problem-solving experience he gains will be invaluable when he begins to face these decisions on his own.

And the time when he will have to do so is just around the corner. Even if your child is just five or six years old, you will be there to control his blood sugars for only a few more years. Once he is in school, he will begin making his own decisions, like what part of his lunch to trade with his best friend. By the time he is age 14 or 15, he will be managing most aspects of his diabetes himself. Start now with a new approach to managing your child's diabetes. Don't try to control his blood sugars. Help him learn how to control them himself.

Deal with Your Fears about Trying This Approach

You may worry that you are being irresponsible or that your child's control will go haywire. But isn't your primary responsibility to prepare your child to solve the daily problems she will face throughout her life with diabetes? You are teaching her the most valuable lesson of all: She can do anything she wants to do, as long as she can figure out how to do it safely. And your child's control will not worsen if she learns to take responsibility for her own care. While she is young, you are still there to veto any particular proposal she might offer, so she is protected in that way. As she gets older and is making more of her decisions independently, she will be better prepared to make them wisely.

It's less likely that she will be left with those all-or-nothing choices of either feeling deprived or letting her blood sugars go where they will.

Continue to Work with Your Older Child

While it may not be your responsibility to control your child's blood sugars, your child is also not responsible for managing her diabetes alone. Even older kids need help and support managing their diabetes at times.

Things can fall between the cracks. The old approach to diabetes care for children was for parents to control everything until the child reached a certain age, usually about 10 years old, and then turn over all responsibility to the child.

Independence in diabetes care was seen as a sign of maturity, a sign the child was taking responsibility for her own diabetes. But research actually shows something quite different. Gary Ingersoll and his colleagues at the University of Indiana conducted a study that tells us a lot about the pitfalls of assuming that just because they are old enough to physically master the required tasks, kids with diabetes will take responsibility for their own care. Ingersoll found that many of the parents he studied withdrew from the process of helping their children adjust insulin doses, but the kids didn't assume the responsibility themselves. Instead, the whole insulin adjustment process simply slipped through the cracks.

Don't focus on age alone. We don't believe that your child's age alone should determine what her part in her diabetes care should be. There is usually a big difference between a child's physical capacity to master a task and the maturity required to do the job on a regular basis. Not recognizing this difference is the source of tremendous frustration for the parents of a child with diabetes: You know she can do her blood sugar tests, so why doesn't she?

In addition, not all kids the same age have the same capacities. Temperament and other individual differences powerfully affect the way children adapt to diabetes or to any other major life challenge.

Also, guidelines don't take into account external stresses or special needs. Family problems, learning disabilities, and a wide range of other factors must be considered when developing a workable diabetes care plan for your family.

Some teenagers seem to adamantly resist taking responsibility for their own diabetes care. If your child acts this way, it is especially important for you to stay as involved as possible and to move slowly as you help her move toward independence. If things get rocky, talk to your child's healthcare team about the possibility of family counseling, preferably with a professional experienced in working with teens who have diabetes.

Balancing the Benefits of Control with the Family's Other Needs

We believe that the most important task facing all parents is to raise emotionally healthy and independent children. That task may be even more important when the child in question has diabetes. After all, the child with diabetes will face special challenges throughout her life. We know that she will need strength, discipline, self-confidence, and great diabetes management skills to deal with the challenges presented by diabetes over the years. If a child grows up observing and participating actively in a balanced and cooperative approach to dealing with diabetes, she is more likely to carry these attitudes and behaviors into adult life. If parents overdo control or give up in despair, the child learns ways of handling her diabetes that will continue to cause her problems throughout her life. Raising a child with diabetes who is healthy in every way is not easy, but it is possible. You need to set personal "good enough" blood sugar goals appropriate to your child's age and ability and to your family's values, supports, and resources. Then you need to help your child learn to take care of herself well enough to achieve them.

Remember, diabetes is not just the child's disease. Diabetes affects the lives of everyone in the family. It affects family activities, routines, and concerns. Families of children whose diabetes is in the best control have two things in common, according to research. First, the children in these families—regardless of their age—have continuing support with diabetes management tasks from their parents. Second, there is not as much conflict in these families as there is in families where kids have less control over their diabetes. You can't totally ignore the gorilla at the symphony we told you about in the book's introduction, but by sharing responsibility for management of diabetes in age-appropriate ways, you can keep that gorilla in its proper place so you can enjoy the process of raising your kids.

THE BOTTOM LINE

1. Blood sugar control is very important, in both the short and long term.
2. Blood sugar goals should be both ambitious and realistic. Goals will change throughout your child's growing-up years.
3. Your job is to help your child learn to control her own blood sugars.
4. The child who learns how to control her own blood sugars will be more independent and emotionally healthy and will achieve better glucose control.
5. A problem-solving approach, based on asking good questions, will help your child learn how to control her own blood sugars.
6. You will have both hits and misses in diabetes management. Learn from both.
7. Begin working on diabetes management and independence with your child at an early age and continue through the teen years.

You're telling me Jared needs to eat six times a day?

6

Why Kids Need Snacks and What to Prepare

Diabetes aside, small frequent feedings work well for most small children.

Jared's mother and father impressed us from the start with their can-do attitude about diabetes. Busy people with lots of commitments, they approach diabetes with the same no-nonsense attitude and organization that they apply to work, sports, and family activities. The day they got the news about Jared's diabetes, they asked a lot of questions and took careful notes as their diabetes team laid out the basics of diabetes care. Amazingly, only one thing about the treatment seemed to bother them: the suggestion that seven-year-old Jared eat snacks between meals and at bedtime.

"I don't believe in eating between meals," Jared's father explained. "My aunts are always noshing on something, and they're way too heavy for their own good. We eat good, substantial meals, and it's always been enough to carry us through. Jared's doing fine, and he hasn't eaten between meals since he started school."

A seven-year-old child who didn't eat between meals sounded like a pretty unique creature to us. Diabetes aside, small frequent feedings work well for most children. Little stomachs coupled with high energy needs mean that most children are ready to eat at least every three or four hours while they're awake. They need more frequent stoking of their energy furnaces—most kids can't last from lunch at noon till dinner at 6 P.M. without eating again. And the 13-hour gap between a 6 P.M. dinner and a 7 A.M. breakfast is more than just about any small stomach can bear. It's not a matter of discipline, as Jared's dad seemed to think. It's a matter of physiology.

We began by explaining that snacks are normal for all kids. We also assured the family that snacks composed of the same good foods they were eating for meals would be a positive nutritional change, not a negative one. Weight gain wouldn't be a problem because we weren't talking about adding three substantial snacks to what Jared was already eating; we just wanted to spread the same amount of food over several meals and snacks. This approach would control his appetite and his blood sugar better.

The Special Role of Snacks in Diabetes

Although snacks are normal for all kids, they can take on special importance in diabetes. The insulin plan needs to be designed so that it allows kids—especially little ones—to eat the snacks they want and need. However, it shouldn't force kids who have outgrown their need for regular snacks to carry boxes of food wherever they go.

When diabetes isn't present, the body puts out short bursts of insulin whenever we eat. Insulin plans that use rapid-acting insulin with meals mimic that natural situation, which works great for adults and older kids who snack infrequently. Taking an extra boost of rapid-acting insulin when you occasionally decide to have a sandwich or a piece of pie in the middle of the day is no big deal. But what about little kids who eat every three hours or so? Giving a shot for every little meal and snack just doesn't make a lot of sense. And sometimes school issues make it a problem for older kids as well. Maybe there's a strict "No Needles" rule, and so Johnny needs to cover lunch with his morning NPH, at least during the school year. In short, many families still have some challenges when it comes to balancing insulin with meals and snacks.

Most people are aware of the role snacks have always played in preventing low blood sugars between meals and during exercise. This is especially important when regular or one of the other longer-acting insulins are used to cover meals. But did you know that snacks can also help prevent *high* blood sugars because they can match the action of those same slower-acting insulins better? And for little kids who still want and need them, snacks can be your secret weapon for avoiding rigid meal plans while still keeping blood sugar under control.

Why Snacks May Be Needed to Prevent Low Blood Sugar

The need for snacks to prevent low blood sugar between meals, overnight, and during exercise is caused by differences between body insulin and some injected insulins. In people who don't have diabetes, the body always produces exactly the right amount of insulin automatically, whenever they decide to eat. They also get small steady amounts of insulin between meals and overnight to keep the blood sugar level perfectly balanced. And they automatically get even less insulin during exercise to help the body release its own sugar supply to provide extra fuel. A great system!

Figure 6.1 shows how much the action of some common injected insulins can differ from that normal picture. The dotted line represents an insulin pattern that's still commonly used for kids: two injections a day of a combination of regular and NPH or Lente insulin. The places where the dotted line is much higher than the solid line (the body's own insulin) are the times when risk for low blood sugar is greatest. Notice that the peak (or greatest action) of the body's insulin is very sharp and occurs right after eating. The peaks of the R and NPH, on the other hand, are less pronounced, last longer, and occur later. Rapid-acting insulin is being used more often to cover meals because it works almost exactly like the body's insulin.

When R and NPH are used for meals, quite a bit of insulin is still around between meals and overnight. If food isn't eaten at those times, the result will be a falling blood sugar level. That pattern can make good sense for little kids who want to eat snacks between meals and at bedtime anyway. But someone who skips a snack on this type of insulin regimen often has problems with lows.

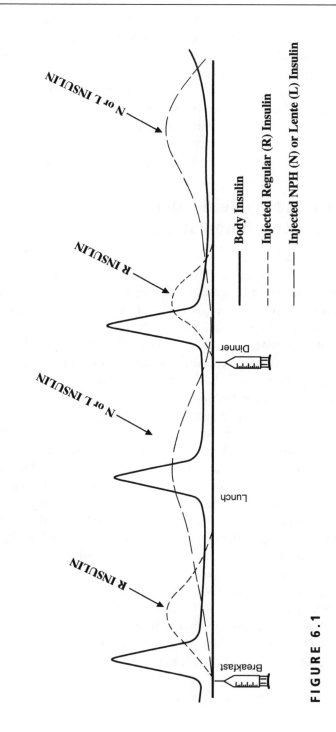

FIGURE 6.1

The same risk for lows can happen during exercise because we're not able to take away insulin that was injected earlier in the day. (*See Chapter 8 for more information about managing exercise.*)

Insulin action depicts *average* times. In fact, there is a tremendous amount of variation in insulin absorption. The longer the insulin lasts, the more variation there is likely to be. Rapid-acting insulin varies very little from day to day in the same person. But regular insulin absorption has been shown to vary between 30 and 40 percent from day to day in the same person using the same injection site! That means 10 units may act like 10 units on one day, 7 on another, and 14 on yet another. The amount of variation is even greater for NPH, Lente, and Ultralente insulins. Keep this in mind on those days when you do everything the same, but your blood sugars make no sense whatsoever. That's why perfect control is not possible with today's tools and why rapid-acting insulin is growing in popularity. It not only acts much more like the body's insulin, it also is more consistent and predictable than the older insulins.

Snacks and Longer-Acting Insulins

Prevent High Blood Sugars after Eating

High blood sugars after meals are a problem for just about everybody with diabetes, at least occasionally. They are less common with rapid-acting insulin, but the blunted peaks of regular, NPH, and Lente insulin also contribute to high blood sugars right after meals. The problem occurs because these insulins don't begin to act until some time after they're injected. Unless there's quite a delay—as much as 45 minutes, or even more—between the shot and the meal, blood sugar from the meal beats the rising level of insulin to the punch. Getting that timing down is hard for most people to do.

The fact is, most people take regular insulin (and the other slower-acting ones) less than 30 minutes before they eat. Sluggish insulin taken that close to the meal just can't handle a whole lot of food at once. That's where snacks can come in. By making meals a bit lighter and moving the difference into snacks, we can better match the action of these particular insulins. This can result in fewer highs and fewer lows, producing more stable blood sugar control.

Relax the Grip of Rigid Meal Plans

One family we know was struggling with their son's variable appetite. Joe was usually eager to eat everything on the exchange meal and snack plan. It's just that he often didn't want it when the plan said he should be eating it. A lot of vigilance went into trying to get Joe to eat the three starch exchanges at breakfast every day, but only one at the morning snack; to not eat fruit with lunch, but always take one fruit exchange with the afternoon snack; to always drink 12 ounces of milk at dinner, but stop at half a cup with the bedtime snack.

The whole family was struggling to stick to the plan, but they followed it only about half of the time. They were tired of fighting over every meal and snack, and who could blame them? Joe liked and needed his snacks, so an insulin plan that eliminated them would not work. And there were issues with the school that made it impossible to consider more daytime injections. But there was another solution.

Think of the Meal Plan in Time Blocks

You can greatly reduce the "rigid-meal-plan blues" associated with set insulin doses and slower insulins by thinking of the meal plan in time blocks instead of as separate meals and snacks. On an R and NPH insulin plan, one meal and one snack are covered by each of the insulins acting during the day. Because of the rather broad peaks of these insulins, the food covered by a given insulin dose can be considered as one block. If we do this, food can be moved back and forth between the meal and snack within a given time block without jeopardizing insulin coverage or blood sugar control.

To help you see exactly how this works, look at the two-injection mixed-insulin plan illustrated in Figure 6.1. On this insulin schedule, the morning regular insulin is expected to last from breakfast until lunch. The broad peak of the morning NPH or Lente probably covers from about lunchtime until dinner. The evening regular insulin covers from dinner until after bedtime, and the evening NPH or Lente acts overnight. If your child takes three injections, he takes his NPH or Lente insulin at bedtime instead of dinnertime. It's still acting overnight, but the peak action takes place closer to dawn than what is shown in the illustration. That's why a third shot is often added when kids are having problems with low blood sugars during the night.

Table 6.1 shows how Joe's unpredictable appetite can be dealt with using the time-block method. The first column shows Joe's usual eating pattern based on his diabetes meal plan and expressed in grams of carbohydrate. The second column shows how it might be divided differently on a day when his appetite is not so hearty at breakfast: The carbohydrate grams not eaten at breakfast could be added to the morning snack. This amounts to almost reversing the order of the snack and the breakfast. If Joe's mother doesn't think he'll be hungry for a full meal at snack time either, she could offer more concentrated sources of carbohydrate. This way he'll get everything he needs in a smaller package: 2/3 cup of grape juice (30 grams of carbohydrate) instead of a cup of strawberries (15 grams of carbohydrate).

The third column shows how Joe's carbohydrate allowance could be divided up on a day when he is feeling extra hungry. Carbohydrate-containing foods are borrowed from the snack in order to satisfy his morning appetite. Food can be moved around within the breakfast-to-lunchtime block in many different combinations. But regardless of exactly when he eats it during the block, he's still getting the same total amount of carbohydrate relative to the same total amount of insulin. In column three, the snack is smaller than usual, because he ate part of it at breakfast. The snack has been filled out with things that don't raise blood sugar, such as raw vegetables and peanuts.

The time-block strategy can also be used when Junior gets himself ousted from the dinner table for acting up. Remember those parent-child job descriptions? The child gets to decide how much he's going to eat of the available food, but he has to follow the family's rules for

TABLE 6.1 Using Time Blocks to Adjust for Changes in Hunger

	Meal Plan	Day 1: Not Hungry	Day 2: Extra Hungry
	57 g carbohydrate	**36 g carbohydrate**	**72 g carbohydrate**
Breakfast	cereal with 4 oz. milk 1/2 banana 1 slice toast 4 oz. milk to drink	cereal with 4 oz. milk 1/2 banana	2 slices toast with peanut butter 1 whole banana 8 oz. milk
	30 g carbohydrate	**51 g carbohydrate**	**15 g carbohydrate**
Morning Snack	8 oz. carton milk 1 cup strawberries	2/3 cup grape juice peanut butter crackers	small can juice celery and peanuts

mealtime behavior. Maybe you had to ask him to leave the table when he made that really rude noise for the third time. If his blood sugar was on the low side before dinner, you might let him take his milk with him when he leaves the table.

Rely on the time-block system to keep things under control. When it comes time for the bedtime snack, add the equivalent of what was missed at dinner. Offer it in a more concentrated form, if you think that's necessary. But the child may be hungry enough by then to just eat the dinner leftovers. If the child needs to eat a substantial bedtime snack because he ate very little at dinner, lay off things you know he doesn't like. Offer some of his preferred foods instead, reducing the chance of another battle.

As it has for many families, the time-block method gave Joe's family a new perspective on how to use their meal plan and made it easier for them to follow the parent and child job descriptions.

What Makes a Good Snack?

Anything that makes a good meal also makes a good snack. To get the best appetite control and most stable blood sugar levels, offer a combination of carbohydrate, protein, and small amounts of fat. Since most of the protein sources we eat—meat, milk, cheese, peanut butter—contain some fat, it's seldom necessary to add fat separately.

Snacks containing only carbohydrate (like fruit, for example) immediately satisfy hunger and release blood sugar quickly, but they won't support blood sugar or control hunger for very long. Snacks composed of only protein and fat (like beef jerky) aren't immediately satisfying and don't provide glucose for insulin coverage. However, the protein and fat tend to provide good long-term appetite control (so the kids are not coming back an hour later for another snack), and the fat slows down the digestion and absorption of starch and sugar, blunting the immediate rise in blood sugar. When you combine carbohydrate, protein, and fat, you get the best of both worlds. Appetite is controlled immediately and for a relatively long time. And you get sustained insulin coverage that begins soon and continues until the next meal or snack.

Table 6.2 shows some of the combinations that work well. Substitute similar foods if these starch/fruit or fat/protein selections aren't appealing. If you and the kids need some new ideas for snacks, we sug-

TABLE 6.2 The Best Snacks Provide Carbohydrate, Fat, and Protein

Carbohydrate Source	Fat/Protein Source
Crackers	String cheese
Bread	Peanut butter
Fresh apple	Reduced-fat cheddar cheese
Dry cereal	Milk
Hot-air popcorn	Sugar-free hot chocolate
Fruit	Cottage cheese
Bread (for sandwich)	Sliced chicken, meat, or cheese
Tortilla	Scrambled egg whites w/salsa

gest getting a copy of *The Joy of Snacks* by Nancy Cooper (American Diabetes Association, Alexandria, VA).

Tips for Bedtime Snacks

Bedtime snacks in diabetes are provided to protect against low blood sugar during sleep, which occurs most commonly between 2 and 3 A.M. This high level of risk is related to four things. First, insulin is much more effective at that time of night because of normal variations in body hormones. Second, it's difficult to adjust NPH or Lente so that the insulin level is low enough between 2 and 3 A.M. (to cut risk for nighttime lows) and also high enough in the early morning hours to avoid high fasting blood sugar. Third, when regular insulin is used to cover the evening meal, it is still strong during the night, increasing the risk for lows. Fourth, most people snack several hours before the time that overnight lows commonly happen. The new long-acting insulin analog, insulin glargine (Lantus), may help reduce the risk for overnight lows. But those still using older insulins for overnight coverage need "time release" bedtime snacks that provide glucose several hours after eating. Some snacks do this and some don't.

To limit falling overnight blood sugar, a snack must contain foods that release their glucose into the bloodstream slowly. As we've said, fats do this pretty well. Fats are digested slowly, so any glucose they produce enters the bloodstream several hours later. But more impor-

TABLE 6.3 Bedtime Snacks Likely to Prevent Overnight Lows

- Pizza and diet soda
- Oatmeal and raisins with milk
- Bean, split pea, lentil, or barley soup
- Bean burrito with cheese
- Sugar-free pudding or yogurt with uncooked cornstarch added

tant, fat slows down the absorption and digestion of carbohydrate. Either way, having some fat in a meal or snack seems to support blood sugar much longer than if carbohydrates are eaten alone. Fats are found in meat, fish, poultry, cheese, milk, yogurt, nuts, and many other foods. Another option for bedtime snacks is starchy foods that are digested very slowly. You may have heard them referred to as Lente carbohydrates or as having a low glycemic index. Our families have had the best results with foods such as oatmeal, barley, pasta, beans, and uncooked cornstarch.

Uncooked cornstarch is one of the "slowest" carbohydrates we know of. It can be stirred into other items, such as yogurt, sugar-free pudding, or peanut butter. Start with a teaspoon of cornstarch (5 grams of carbohydrate) and increase a teaspoon at a time up to a tablespoon, or three teaspoons, until blood sugars stay in a desirable range overnight. You'll need to use those 2 to 3 A.M. blood tests to see how your experiments with different bedtime snacks are working. Table 6.3 has some examples of specific snacks that have worked well for children who were having problems with low blood sugar in the middle of the night.

But trying to manage food so carefully is not the only answer. Talk to your team about how your insulin regimen might reduce or elim-inate this problem at the source. One common solution is to move the dinnertime NPH or Lente insulin to bedtime, which may help move the peak closer to dawn, where it causes less risk for lows and may do a bet-ter job of controlling fasting blood sugar. Of course, this means another injection, but if that's acceptable, it can work pretty well. For very young children with early bedtimes, Mom or Dad can give the NPH or Lente at their own bedtime. Many children won't even wake up for it.

Switching from regular to rapid-acting insulin for meals often results in fewer problems with overnight lows. Another option is switching to insulin glargine for background insulin. And, of course, the insulin pump can help eliminate this problem, with its ability to so precisely provide low levels of insulin overnight. But even with glargine and the pump, nighttime testing—at least occasionally—is important to make sure lows aren't happening during the night.

But whether your child eats a bedtime snack because he wants to, he needs to, or both, don't forget to have him brush his teeth. Diabetes is associated with a much higher risk for gum disease and cavities, so good dental hygiene is especially important.

Timing of Snacks

By controlling the timing and the type of food for snacks, you increase the chances that they will satisfy your child's hunger and help with blood sugar control. Midway between meals is best for most kids. If snacks are available too soon after a meal, the child may refuse them because he's not hungry yet. Or it may encourage him to eat less at the meal, holding out for more preferred foods at snack time. Having the snack halfway between the meals makes it more likely that he'll be hungry for the snack—but not too hungry. Delaying snack time until a child is famished raises the likelihood of fussiness and arguments.

Spreading meals and snacks out pretty evenly through the day also provides good insulin coverage, reducing the likelihood of extreme highs and lows in the blood sugar. Two snacks are okay if it's a really long stretch between meals. If this happens, make the last snack completely or mostly carbohydrate—fruit, juice, or crackers, for example. These foods are not as likely to stick around long enough to interfere with the child's appetite for the coming meal. They also have a somewhat shorter effect on the blood sugar, which is good because you're probably going to be checking the blood sugar before the next meal.

Sometimes a snack cannot be eaten at the planned time. Maybe the drive home took an extra 45 minutes because of a traffic jam. Or maybe the teacher kept the whole class after school. Perhaps your child forgot to take his snack with him when he went out bike riding and returned home famished less than an hour before dinner. Things happen—it's called life. What you do about it, of course, depends on the situation. What's his blood sugar? How long is it until the next meal? Is the child hungry?

Here are some options. If the delayed snack produced low blood sugar, treat the low blood sugar first. Then give the planned snack. Depending on how low the glucose fell, you may need to give more than was originally planned for the snack. If the blood sugar is in the desired range, just go ahead and give the snack. But if the next meal is coming up fairly soon, you may want to eliminate some or all of the fat and protein from the snack to help make sure that the child will be hungry for the coming meal. If his blood glucose is high but he still wants a snack, you can reduce the amount of carbohydrate in the snack to prevent driving the blood sugar up even higher.

What if Blood Sugars Are Too High after Snacks?

You can deal with blood sugars that are consistently above your child's target range before a meal in several ways, depending on your preferences and the cause of the high readings. First, make sure that you're not testing too close to the snack. (There are, undoubtedly, differences in your goals for after-meal and before-meal blood sugars. For example, many people try to keep before-meal blood sugars between 80 and 120 mg/dl [4–7 mmol] or 80 and 140 mg/dl [4–8 mmol]. Goals for after-meal blood sugars are more likely to be less than 160 [9 mmol], or 180 [10 mmol].) If a test is done less than two hours after eating, it will be on the high side, but hopefully not higher than the after-meal goal. This can happen even if the total amount of food is well matched by the insulin dose. You may want to change the timing of the snack based on the insulin peak.

If the snack was eaten more than a couple of hours before a high test, you need to decide whether the situation calls for changing the food or changing the insulin. If you feel that the total amount of food in the time block (breakfast plus the morning snack, for example) is right for your child's appetite, one option is to increase the insulin dose working at that time to better cover that amount of food. (*See Chapter 4 for some general guidelines on insulin adjustments for high blood sugar and for variations in eating.*) You could also cut down on the amount of carbohydrate by either moving a starch or fruit serving into the previous meal or reducing the total amount of carbohydrate. This can be accomplished by simply eliminating a serving of a high-carbohydrate food or by substituting foods that have less effect on blood sugar. The best approach depends on your child's appetite and food preferences, as well as his overall nutritional intake.

For example, eight-year-old Linda's blood sugar had been around 200 mg/dl before lunch for three days in a row. She had her snack about 10 A.M. and lunch at 12:30 P.M., so the reading probably wasn't related to testing too soon after the snack. She was having two starch servings, one fruit, and one milk at breakfast and two more starches and a milk at her morning snack. She and her mom talked about whether she would like to make the snack smaller and eat more at breakfast or just cut down a bit. She said breakfast was just right. She didn't want to make that any bigger. She didn't really want to make the snack any smaller either. She didn't think one starch and a milk would be enough to carry her until lunch. Linda and her mom decided to change her snack by replacing one of the starches in her snack with some protein. This would provide less carbohydrate, but about the same total amount of food. She could have a cracker and cheese snack pack or half a peanut butter sandwich with her milk. She was happy with the change. It satisfied her appetite and improved her blood sugar before lunch as well.

Occasionally, a child will want to eat such a substantial snack that an extra dose of insulin is needed to cover it. This is most often an issue with the after-school snack. Regardless of which insulin is covering the afternoon time period, there may not be enough around by 3 or 4 o'clock in the afternoon to handle a really big snack. Some kids are so active after school with play or sports that this is never an issue. They run off whatever they eat. Other kids are famished when they get home from school and want to eat everything in sight. If your youngster has high blood sugars following really substantial snacks, a small extra insulin bolus may be needed to keep things in control. The dose will probably be smaller than what you would give for the same amount of food if it was eaten at a meal, because there may still be some insulin remaining from the previous injection. If your child is having this type of problem, be sure to check with your healthcare provider before adding any extra insulin shots to her schedule. Caution is doubly important if there's going to be another shot in a few hours at the next meal. If the child resists adding another shot, try changing the composition of the snack. Less carbohydrate with more protein, fat, or fiber may produce better blood sugar control, eliminating the need for a booster insulin injection.

One young patient named Geri liked to have a sandwich, a bag of chips, milk, and a cookie after school. This was basically a second lunch, and because it came late in the afternoon, the remainder of her morning NPH just wasn't getting the job done. We tried increasing the morning dose, but that just tended to make Geri low before she got out of school. Next we tried a two-unit booster of rapid-acting insulin before she ate her snack. That wouldn't have been anywhere near enough insulin for that amount of food at a regular meal. Even so, it worked great for her afternoon snack because it was teaming up with her morning NPH.

Getting Kids to Carry Snacks

When children are small, most of their snacks are eaten at home. But even toddlers will occasionally go to the park or other places and need to carry snacks along. And older kids will be taking most of their snacks away from home. Questions arise about where to stash them, how to carry them, and how to get kids to carry their own.

Avoid becoming that well known (at least in diabetes circles) superhero: Simple Sugar Woman (or Man)! You know, the one who leaps over tall benches full of Little Leaguers in a single bound to give Johnny a box of juice when she sees him looking pale.

Carrying his own snacks (and other diabetes supplies) puts your child in a position to handle this kind of problem on his own and helps him learn to control his own blood sugars. Mom and Dad simply won't be there to do it forever, so it's important for the child to take on this responsibility in age-appropriate steps. The youngest children may simply wear a backpack that was filled by another family member. The next step might be helping to choose the specific foods to include. At some point, the child can become part of the kitchen brigade, helping with the actual food preparation. And finally, the child can plan, prepare, and tote his own snacks, touching base with Mom and Dad on occasion to check out the details.

For children who develop diabetes at a very young age, it seems to work quite well to make them responsible for carrying their own snacks from the start. Most toddlers and preschoolers enjoy having their own colorful pack or decorated lunch bag (they can decorate the paper ones themselves). They'll probably get in the habit of carrying one if it is presented matter-of-factly. Of course, it's a good idea for

Mom and Dad also to carry or stash a backup supply for emergencies, at least in the early years.

Older kids can keep snacks and their other diabetes supplies in the same kinds of book bags, gym bags, and other packs that their friends use. Diabetes supplies don't have to look like diabetes supplies when they leave home. And if it takes a cooler to hold all the food needed to get Junior through the day— run, don't walk, back to your team for some help with that insulin plan!

Many parents we've worked with routinely include enough snack food for a friend or friends when preparing a snack for their child. This puts the snacking in a much more positive light; it becomes an opportunity to share with friends rather than a requirement to do something that sets your child apart as different.

What if, in spite of all your support and low-key encouragement, your child consistently refuses or "forgets" to carry snacks or other diabetes needs? Clearly, safety demands that you step in. Insulin, food, and blood-testing supplies need to be handy. Use questioning, experimentation, and problem-solving (as described in Chapter 5) to develop mutually acceptable solutions. Address specific situations one at a time (*see Chapter 14 for some tips on how diabetes tasks can be broken down into many separate steps*). Your child may not yet be willing to take complete responsibility for carrying snacks or supplies, but you may be able to agree on some small steps toward that eventual goal to get him started. Good luck!

What if He Simply Won't Eat a Snack?

Children will sometimes refuse to eat a snack that's needed to cover insulin. This refusal can be direct ("I'm not going to eat it!") or indirect (snack foods found in the bottom of the wastebasket after school). Giving the child who balks at the regimen a chance to refuse a snack can help defuse the situation. It's also consistent with your respective job descriptions: You provide it, he decides whether or not to eat it. There are several possible outcomes. The child may have no ill effects at all from skipping the snack. This is most likely if his blood sugar was running high to start with. If his blood sugar was fairly normal, the child may start to get mildly low and have a change of heart, finding his missing appetite in a hurry. Or if the blood sugar was on the low side to begin with, the child may go even lower and really need treatment.

That's okay, especially if you're in a controlled setting, such as your home. Remember, people learn from their experiences. It is responsible to allow children to learn the consequences of their diabetes-related behaviors firsthand, in a safe environment. If you let this happen at home without a lot of angst, the child can learn for himself why snacks are important for him at this time. But don't reinforce this lesson with a lot of "I told you so's." This may put the child on the defensive, which could detract from any learning that has taken place.

Your judgment here is crucial. The same approach would not be a good idea if you knew your kid was heading off on a long bike ride or was set to compete in a sports event; these are not controlled, safe environments. (Such circumstances call for the kind of family problem solving described in Chapter 5.) With that approach, you and your child can work together to find a way for him to get what he wants—to go for the bike ride or compete in the sport event—while you get what you want—for your child to be safe during these activities.

If you have thought of snacks as a burdensome part of your child's care in the past, we hope we have given you a new perspective. Snacks are natural to small children. With certain insulin regimens, they can also help smooth out blood sugar control, blunting after-meal highs and preventing between-meal lows. And for those following defined meal plans, they can free you from some of the plan's rigidity. Using the time-block method can help keep food and insulin in sync despite your kid's variable appetite and personal quirks.

THE BOTTOM LINE

For all kids:

1. Small children need snacks because of high energy needs and small stomach capacities.

For kids with diabetes:

1. Rapid-acting insulin at meals reduces the diabetes-related need for snacks.

2. With other insulins, snacks help prevent low blood sugar between meals and overnight.

3. Snacks help prevent high blood sugar by matching insulin demand more closely to the action of regular, NPH, and Lente used to cover meals.

4. Snacks containing carbohydrate, protein, and fat do the best job of controlling appetite and smoothing out blood sugars.

5. Food from meals and snacks in the same insulin time block can be moved around to match appetite and control blood sugars.

6. Work on the insulin plan with your team to reduce risk for overnight lows.

7. Include fat or "Lente carbohydrate" in bedtime snacks to help support blood sugar all night long.

I could feel my blood sugar getting lower and lower, but I didn't have anything to eat with me . . .

7

Preventing and Treating Low Blood Sugar

Lindy was 17 and totally against anything that would "expose" her diabetes to her friends. She refused to take a lunchtime shot at school. She spent her own money to get the smallest blood sugar meter she could find and kept it at the bottom of her backpack and only used it (in a bathroom stall) if she was feeling really bad. Her diabetes educator suggested that she always carry something to treat low blood sugar, but Lindy insisted she would be fine because she always carried money to buy a soft drink or candy.

So the educator was quite surprised when Lindy showed up for her appointment one day with a supply of crackers, candy, and some boxed juice. Lindy laughed when she explained that she and a friend had been trapped in an elevator at school for nearly two hours a few days earlier. The elevator clunked to a stop just before lunch. As the lunch hour ticked by, Lindy could feel her blood sugar getting lower and lower. And, of course, the change she carried to buy food wasn't doing

Eating a moldy cheese sandwich convinced Lindy that it was a good idea to carry food with her.

her any good in that elevator. After trying to hide the situation for a while, she finally told her friend what was happening and asked if she had anything to eat.

"Sure. I've still got my lunch from a couple of days ago. You're welcome to it." Eating a moldy cheese sandwich convinced Lindy, in a way that advice never could, that it was a good idea to carry food with her.

Lindy was hardly alone in her problems with low blood sugar. A child with diabetes commonly averages at least one low blood sugar episode a week. Fortunately, most of these are fairly mild, but even the mildest low is unpleasant. More severe episodes can be embarrassing, scary, and even dangerous. You may also know low blood sugar by the terms "insulin reaction," "hypo," or simply, "reaction." But by any name, it means the same thing: trouble.

Hypoglycemia can interfere with your child's thinking, making mental tasks—like doing schoolwork or even getting the food she needs to treat herself—difficult or impossible. It can also make physical activities, such as riding a bicycle or driving a car, hazardous. When someone is really afraid of lows, however, they sometimes let blood sugars run high all the time. That might feel safe at the moment but increases the risk for complications in the long run. Low blood sugar is a big deal for both you and your child.

In fact, many parents tell us that hypoglycemia (both the reality and the fear of it) has a powerful negative effect on families. Arguments often arise when parents push their kids to be responsible—to carry food, wear a medical I.D., or let people know how to help if they go low, for example. And kids, for their part, vigorously resist these precautions.

Low Blood Sugar Defined

What exactly do we mean by hypoglycemia? Some people define lows solely by blood glucose level, such as less than 60 mg/dl (3.3 mmol), but we don't. Just the number isn't enough. Some people do fine with a blood sugar of 60 mg/dl, while others clearly feel hypoglycemic at 80 mg/dl (4.4 mmol). We say a child is hypoglycemic when her blood sugar is low enough to cause her to feel or act hypoglycemic, but she recovers when her sugar level comes back up. Hypoglycemia can cause a variety of symptoms, and they may not relate to the actual blood sugar level.

Symptoms of Hypoglycemia

The common symptoms of hypoglycemia fall into three categories: physical, mental, and emotional. You've probably observed all three in your child at various times. People experience symptoms of hypoglycemia at different blood sugar levels. What's more, the same person may have different symptoms on different days: She may feel anxious and sweaty one day when her blood sugar is 80 mg/dl (4.4 mmol) and not have any symptoms at all a few days later at a blood sugar of 40 mg/dl (2.2 mmol).

Physical symptoms. Physical symptoms of low blood sugar include lightheadedness or dizziness, poor coordination, pounding heart, trembling, and sweating. Some of these symptoms (including the last three) are not actually caused by the low blood sugar; they are caused by counterregulatory hormones that the body releases to protect itself from going too low. These hormones cause the liver to release stored sugar into the bloodstream. The term "counterregulatory" refers to the fact that these hormones work opposite insulin in regulating the blood sugar level. Insulin lowers blood sugar. The counterregulatory hormones—epinephrine (also called adrenaline), glucagon, cortisol, and growth hormone—raise it. Whenever your child's sugar level falls to a certain point (usually, but not always, about 50 mg/dl or 2.8 mmol), the body releases these hormones to bring it back up.

The body releases adrenaline when we are in a stressful situation, a reaction also known as the fight-or-flight response. The physical symptoms of low blood sugar—shaking, trembling, a rapid heart beat, anxiety—and those of the fight-or-flight stress response are identical. In fact, although these symptoms may be reliable signs that your child is hypoglycemic, they are not a direct result of low blood sugar itself but of her body's efforts to counteract the hypoglycemia.

Other symptoms you might notice when your child is low include visual disturbances (double vision, seeing spots, even temporary partial blindness), sudden hunger, a headache, a stomach ache, or sudden and severe fatigue. We have been amazed at the variety of symptoms children describe: One will tell us her hands feel numb, while another feels as if everyone around her is moving farther and farther away. Many can't provide any better description of how they feel other than to say they feel funny.

Mental symptoms. If your child's blood sugar level goes really low, her brain becomes starved for glucose and can't work right. The mental symptoms of low blood sugar include difficulty concentrating, clumsiness, spaciness, dizziness, confusion, headache, slurred or slow speech, and fatigue. If your child shows any of these signs of moderate to severe hypoglycemia, immediate action must be taken. They indicate that the blood sugar is getting low enough to lead to loss of consciousness or a seizure.

Emotional symptoms. You've probably noticed that low blood sugar affects your child's mood, too. When she is hypoglycemic she may get irritable or act funny. Parents often pick up on hypoglycemia by subtle (or not so subtle) changes in mood or personality. One father we know gently suggests that his son test his blood sugar whenever he suspects the child is low. If his son reacts angrily with a statement like, "Leave me alone. I don't need to test my blood sugar!" he replies, "You're absolutely right, you don't need to test. You can go straight to the orange juice." Since the boy is usually easygoing, his dad has learned that the most likely cause for an angry outburst is hypoglycemia.

Levels of Hypoglycemia

Mild hypoglycemia. When your child has mild hypoglycemia, her symptoms generally do not interfere much with her normal activities. You or she may notice a change in her thought processes, but it may not be apparent to people who don't know her well. These episodes may be uncomfortable or upsetting, but most often they are only a nuisance and respond quickly to treatment.

Moderate hypoglycemia. With moderate hypoglycemia, there is a more obvious problem, in the form of confusion, inappropriate behavior, or both. But she is still alert enough to treat her own low blood sugar or to let you know that she needs help. Recovery typically takes a bit longer than with the mild form.

Severe hypoglycemia. When hypoglycemia is severe, your child is so confused that she cannot treat herself or get help. She may even have a seizure or fall into a coma. If your child has ever had such an episode, you know how frightening severe hypoglycemia can be. These episodes are often more upsetting for parents, since the child is often uncon-scious and unaware of what's occurring. A child may feel tired and washed out for quite some time after a severe low sugar reaction, even after the blood sugar is back to normal.

Symptoms Aren't a Foolproof Guide

Everyone is different. Unfortunately, symptoms are not an absolutely reliable sign of hypoglycemia. The signs that your child is hypo-glycemic may be completely different from another child's; some symptoms may even be unique to them. One seven-year-old child we knew had a lot of problems with hypoglycemia, but he didn't have any of the common symptoms to warn him that he was getting low. Then one day he finally discovered a reliable sign: He got a tickle in the back of his throat. He might be the only person with this symptom, but it worked for him, and that's what matters.

Sometimes kids feel low when they are not. You may also notice times that your child feels hypoglycemic, but when you test, she is actually not low. It could be that she is trying to talk herself (or you) into believing she needs something to eat. But it could also be the result of her blood sugar coming down very rapidly from a high level, yet still not being low. The body seems to take a rapid drop in blood sugar as a sign of developing hypoglycemia, and it responds by releasing counter-regulatory hormones as a protective measure. Your child could also simply be anxious and confusing the symptoms of anxiety with those of hypoglycemia. Furthermore, some children can't feel any real differ-ence between the symptoms of low blood sugar and those of high blood sugar.

Symptoms can vary over time—and may even disappear. Relying on symptoms is also tricky because your child's hypoglycemic symptoms may vary over time, even from day to day, sometimes even disappear-ing almost completely. If your child doesn't feel low until her blood sugar level is well below 50 mg/dl (2.8 mmol), waiting for symptoms could mean that she would be in serious trouble before anything could be done about it.

A child who repeatedly feels no obvious symptoms until her blood sugar is less than 50 mg/dl (2.8 mmol) has quite a serious problem: She has lost the early physical warning signs that her blood sugar is dropping dangerously low. This state, called hypoglycemia unawareness (or more precisely, diminished awareness), can develop if your child has several episodes of low blood sugar in a short period of time. It happens because the body adapts to frequent lows by becoming better at getting along on smaller amounts of blood sugar. This adaptation keeps the body from releasing counterregulatory hormones when blood sugar is moderately low, and the early-warning system fails to work.

In children, this situation is usually temporary, yet it can still be quite a problem, since it makes it harder to recognize and treat lows before they become serious. The best way to restore normal early-warning symptoms is to avoid all hypoglycemia for a few days by running blood sugars a bit higher than usual.

Even though your child's symptoms are not a foolproof guide to his or her blood sugar level, recognizing them is still key to avoiding serious problems. Both you and your child need to be alert for her own particular symptoms. When watchfulness is coupled with frequent and timely blood testing, you will identify many developing lows before they get serious. The rule is, if in doubt, test.

Causes and Prevention of Hypoglycemia

When your child's blood sugar is low, the culprit is almost always one or more of the following: near-normal control, too much insulin, too little food, or too much exercise. Older kids can also have low blood sugar problems from drinking alcohol or, in girls, from the hormonal changes of the menstrual cycle.

Near-Normal Control

As we have seen, keeping your child's blood sugars as close to normal as possible can increase her risk of hypoglycemia. That's because there's much less margin for error if you are aiming for near-normal levels than if blood sugar is higher. The DCCT intensive treatment group had three times as much hypoglycemia as participants who practiced conventional treatment. However, the DCCT was conducted solely with regular insulin, and we now have good evidence that intensive treatment with the rapid-acting analogs is associated with much less hypoglycemia than intensive treatment with regular insulin. Still, any time blood sugars are maintained near normal, there will be a substantial risk for lows, requiring extra watchfulness.

Preventing problems. Because the risk of hypoglycemia increases when you try for tight blood sugar control, you and your child have to work hard to anticipate and prevent problems. You can't do this all the time, and your child won't always cooperate, but there are strategies that can help. First, be aware of "near-lows." If your child always tends to run 70 to 90 mg/dl (3.9 to 5 mmol) at some particular time, once in a while her blood sugar will be 50 mg/dl at that time, and she will be in trouble. So try not to cut it too close. A bit less insulin or a bit more food can correct a pattern of near-lows, reducing the risk of hypoglycemia.

Restoring hypoglycemia awareness. Next, ease up a little on glucose goals when the situation calls for it. If your child has been having a lot of lows, for example, don't push so hard to keep her blood sugars down, at least for a few days. As we've mentioned, a vicious cycle can start: Low blood sugars reduce your child's ability to detect low blood sugars, thus causing more lows; however, even a few days free from hypoglycemia can restore the body's ability to detect low blood sugar. Frequent lows—especially severe ones—can also deplete the body's supplies of stored sugar. If this happens, the body can no longer protect itself against serious lows because this safety net has been lost. Eating enough food, taking the right amount of insulin, and avoiding severe lows allows the body to rebuild its stores of sugar as well as its capacity to recognize lows.

Special situations. You may also want to ease up for certain situations in which low blood sugar would be a real problem: an athletic event, driving a car, or a camping trip, for instance. This can be a tricky business, of course. These same stressful situations could push blood sugars higher, which creates its own acute problems. Being aware and flexible and gathering enough blood sugar data can help you navigate the course successfully.

Very young children. Finally, you may need to adjust your goals for glycemic control if your child is younger than seven years of age. This is important for two reasons. First, until about age seven, your child's brain is still developing, and she needs glucose for this purpose. Low blood sugars during this period can interfere with brain and nervous system development. Second, a very young child may be less able than an older child to let you know when she is getting hypoglycemic. You may not be able to distinguish the signs of low blood sugar from normal fussiness or sleepiness. When a very young child is low and you don't know it, you may not be able to treat her hypoglycemia in a timely manner.

Too Much Insulin

From one perspective, having too much insulin for the current need causes all hypoglycemia. (We will talk later in this chapter about how food and exercise can tilt the scales toward low blood sugar.) Various insulins and therapy options can make it more or less likely that your child will sometimes have too much insulin on board. To begin with, different insulins are related to lows at different times of the day, so the time of day that low blood sugar occurs can point to the particular insulin that is causing it. For example, too much morning regular insulin is especially likely to make your child low from about mid-morning to lunchtime. And too much morning NPH or Lente insulin can make her low from late morning until dinnertime. Early morning (1 to 3 A.M.) hypoglycemia can be caused by too much NPH or Lente insulin at dinner or bedtime, but nighttime lows can also be related to regular insulin taken with the evening meal. No insulin is free of risk for lows, but the more closely the insulin plan mimics the body's insulin levels, the less likely it is that lows will occur.

Absorption problems. Hypoglycemia can also be caused by uneven or changed absorption of insulin. Uneven absorption is a characteristic of injected insulin and is pretty much uncontrollable. Ultralente insulin tends to be more variable than Lente, Lente more unpredictable than NPH, and NPH more variable than regular insulin. And regular insulin is more variable than any of the analog insulins (Novolog, Humalog, and Lantus). Regular insulin is known to vary at least 30 to 40 percent in absorption from day to day in the same person. Eliminating or at least greatly reducing the variability of insulin absorption is one of the great things about the analog insulins.

Insulin absorption can also be changed by various factors. If your child exercises a part of her body into which she has just injected insulin (such as running, after injecting into the thigh), faster absorption may trigger low blood sugar. Absorption can also be speeded up by heat (such as sitting in a hot tub or warm bath, taking a shower, or sunbathing), bringing on low blood sugar because the insulin peaks earlier than usual. Even changing the injection site can contribute to insulin variability and blood sugar swings.

New insulin bottle. Because insulin slowly loses its strength once the bottle is opened, lows can also happen when people start a new bottle. If a bottle lasts a very long time (as it does in kids who take tiny insulin doses), the insulin may weaken quite a bit. You might be increasing dosages to make up for the loss of strength, but taking the same dose from a new, full-strength bottle of insulin can push the blood sugar too low. Also, if your child switches to a more purified insulin, or from mixed species to single species, or to human insulin from animal insulin, her blood sugars may dip if the same doses are used. Anytime you switch insulins, it's a good idea to do more frequent blood testing so you can make any adjustments to the dosage as quickly as possible.

When your child has several episodes of low blood sugar in a row at the same time of day, you'll have to cut down her dose on your own or with the help of your healthcare provider. Since your goal is to help your child learn to control her own blood sugars, talk to her about the reasoning behind any changes. Even children too young to make such decisions on their own can begin to absorb some of it, and being included in the process will build her confidence and competence for managing when she's on her own.

To avoid such problems entirely, try not to keep a bottle, cartridge, or prefilled insulin pen in use for longer than the manufacturer recommends. The exact time period varies from about a week for some prefilled insulin pens to around a month for a bottle. The countdown begins on the day you first pierce the bottle top or cartridge with a syringe or needle. Check the package insert to find the exact time for the insulins your child uses. Unopened insulin kept in the refrigerator will stay at full strength until the expiration date printed on the box.

Tools for Preventing Lows

A certain amount of extra insulin between meals and overnight can't be avoided with most of the available insulins (regular, NPH, Lente, and Ultralente) because of the way they are absorbed and used by the body. (*See Figure 6.1, which compares the action of injected insulins with that of the body's own insulin.*) But some tools can help produce insulin levels that are more like the body's.

Pumps. One tool that can reduce excess insulin is the insulin pump. Pumps give out insulin in small, precise amounts throughout the day and night, which reduces the risk for hypoglycemia. But for a variety of reasons, pumps haven't traditionally been used much for younger kids. For one thing, they're expensive. Health insurance often covers the cost, but for a family without coverage, finances can be a barrier. Another reason is that there are still relatively few healthcare providers who have had much experience using pumps with this age group. There are pediatric diabetes programs around the country that have had great success using pumps in teens, school-age kids, and even babies and toddlers, but they are the exception, rather than the rule. If there is a diabetes team in your area that is skilled in the use of pumps, it might be worth considering—both for the pump's ability to lower hypoglycemia risk and for its greater flexibility for meals and exercise.

Studies show that pumps can improve A1C levels and reduce the risk of hypoglycemia in adolescents without adversely affecting their quality of life. In fact, teens using pumps reported they had less trouble coping with the daily demands of diabetes than teens who were taking shots. In children too young to manage their pumps independently, pumps have been used at night, which seemed to improve overnight control. And there are now pumps with "lock out" and remote control features that make them secure, even in babies and toddlers. Pumps are a lot of work and, even with insurance coverage, cost more, but many families feel they are well worth it.

Pens. Insulin pens are the most common insulin delivery device in many parts of the world outside of the United States. In fact, we are last among all the industrialized countries in pen use. The pens, which have become popular over the last two decades primarily because of their convenience and accuracy, come in two forms: prefilled and reusable. Prefilled pens have an insulin reservoir built in, and the whole pen is discarded when it is empty. Refillable pens use insulin cartridges; the cartridge is discarded and replaced when it is empty. Both types of pens use fine-gauge needles that are screwed onto the pen barrel. Their ability to accurately deliver small insulin doses makes them a natural for children with diabetes. In addition, their convenience encourages people to take their insulin at just the right time, further reducing hypoglycemia risk.

Insulin Analogs. Insulin analogs are also known as designer insulins. One type of analog is rapid-acting insulin. There are two of these on the market. They are almost exactly like body insulin but have been slightly altered to act in ways that improve therapy. Rapid-acting insulin analogs act faster than regular insulin and are a lot like the body's own meal-related doses of insulin. They peak quickly and then disappear quickly as well, reducing the risk for low blood sugars between meals and overnight. The brands of rapid-acting analog currently available are: Humalog (Eli Lilly), and Novolog (Novo Nordisk). Humalog came on the U.S. market in 1996 and Novolog in 2001.

Lantus, or insulin glargine (Aventis), is a long-acting insulin analog that has virtually no peak in most people. It is usually used once daily, at bedtime. In clinical trials, adults and children using Lantus for their background insulin needs had less hypoglycemia, especially at night, when compared with people using NPH, Lente, or Ultralente.

Facts about Lantus, Humalog, and Novolog are summarized in Table 7.1. Analogs won't totally eliminate low blood sugar, of course, but they can reduce the risk, particularly when used in combination.

Too Little Food

A mismatch between food and insulin, either in amount or in timing, is less of an issue for kids who adjust doses for food. But for those on unchanging doses or nonphysiologic insulin plans, skipping meals or snacks, delaying them for more than a few minutes, or eating less than usual can lead to low blood sugars.

When a child takes her premeal insulin and then refuses to eat, parents begin pressuring the child to eat, fearing severe low blood sugar and a frantic call to 911. But as we discussed earlier, pressuring almost always results in kids actually eating less, not more. It's best to prevent such situations from happening, but if one does arise, we recommend you let your child eat reasonably healthy that suits her and will supply the amount of carbohydrate that's in the usual meal.

Try this. Mom gives five-year-old Johnny four units of regular insulin to cover his usual evening meal containing about 75 grams of carbohy-

TABLE 7.1 Facts about Analog Insulins

Rapid-Acting Analogs

- A rapid-acting version of human insulin that is similar to the body's own insulin. Begins to work almost immediately; peaks in about an hour; lasts only about three hours.
- Two brands available: Humalog from Eli Lilly and Novolog from Novo Nordisk.
- Used with meals in place of regular insulin. NPH, Lantus, Lente, or Ultralente insulin must be used with rapid-acting analogs to meet basal (between meals and overnight) insulin needs in type 1 diabetes.
- Doses are matched to meal composition. If switching from regular, doses will be unit-for-unit or less.
- Reduces risk for hypoglycemia between meals and overnight because it is shorter acting.
- Provides excellent control of after-meal blood sugars when taken with the meal. Regular insulin tends to lead to elevated after-meal blood sugars when taken with meals.
- No need to test and inject 30 to 45 minutes before eating. All care can be done right at mealtime.

Long-Acting Analog

- A long-acting version of human insulin that lasts for about 24 hours and does not have a peak in most people.
- Brand name is Lantus, from Aventis Pharmaceuticals.
- Usually taken once a day, at bedtime. Cannot be mixed with other insulins.
- Used in place of NPH, Lente, and Ultralente to meet background insulin needs.
- Most people have fewer lows with Lantus than with other background insulins because of its predictable absorption and absence of a peak.

drate (three starch exchanges and one milk, one vegetable, and one fruit exchange). But Johnny played hard this afternoon. Tired and cranky, he takes one look at the tuna-noodle casserole she made and starts to cry. "That's yucky," he wails. "I don't want any." Since his blood sugar was 90 mg/dl (5 mmol) before supper, Mom knows he's going to need something pretty soon to cover the insulin and the extra activity. A wise woman, she avoids getting into a shouting match over the casserole. "I'm sorry you don't like what we're having. We've got some other things on the table that you like. What looks good to you?"

Johnny may choose the bread that's on the table for dinner. Mom can throw in some peanut butter to sweeten the pot, if that will increase the likelihood of the bread being eaten. With milk and fruit, it should be possible to replace the 75 grams of carbohydrate without too much fuss.

Or try this. If the child has a really poor appetite, offer more concentrated sources of carbohydrate so you can cover the insulin with less total food volume. This is no time to offer the reduced-calorie cranberry juice cocktail (1 cup = 15 grams of carbohydrate); instead, go for grape juice or a fruit nectar (1/3 cup = 15 grams of carbohydrate). Skip the popcorn (3 cups = 15 grams of carbohydrate) and go for a biscuit or muffin (1 small muffin = 15 grams of carbohydrate). Basically, offer choices that are both well liked and fairly concentrated.

Avoid pressuring the child to eat. It's counterproductive. Also, avoid offering sweets *only* at times like this. It might encourage the child to act up in order to get things that aren't available at other times. (*See Chapter 5 for tips on incorporating sweets into meals.*) And remember, the sugar in chocolate and other candies containing a lot of fat may be absorbed more slowly than that in fat-free candies, so they might not be the best choice for times like this. However, what works best to raise low blood glucose is quite individual. If one thing doesn't work, try another. One two-year-old we know flatly refused to eat or drink anything when she was low. Her mom finally discovered that if she just set three candy-coated chocolate drops in front of the little girl, without trying to get her to eat them, the child would slowly and cautiously stick one in her mouth. This actually raised her blood sugar enough that Mom could get her to drink some juice. Creativity and an open mind can work wonders.

Some of the insulins that are used to cover meals (regular, NPH, Lente, and Ultralente) are active for longer periods than the body's own insulin, so your child doesn't have to eat exactly the right amount at every meal and snack. If dinner is on the light side, add the missing carb to the next snack—just make sure it's more concentrated in carbohydrate and something she's sure to like. (*Refer to Chapter 6 to see how moving food between a meal and a snack can help you deal with variations in your child's appetite.*)

If this mealtime dilemma happens a lot, you could give the insulin after your child has eaten. This tactic is not uncommon with infants, toddlers, and preschoolers whose eating may be unpredictable or who go on food jags. The rapid-acting analogs are perfect for this; regular won't provide the best blood sugar control, but even taking regular after the meal is probably better than turning dinnertime into a donnybrook.

Another way to reduce hypoglycemia risk in little kids who are refusing to eat is to reduce by half the insulin dose that covers the problem meal. Try this for a few days. With so much less insulin, you can feel relaxed about letting her eat as little as she wants. This can break the cycle and allow you to readjust insulin as her eating habits get back to normal. Once you find a way to prevent food refusal from becoming a scene, she will probably stop doing it. Remember, kids don't willingly starve themselves. They generally only get really balky about food over long periods of time if it's turned into a battle of wills.

Too Much Exercise

Consider the difficulties of managing the effects of unplanned, prolonged, or high-intensity physical activity on blood sugar. And what child doesn't play this way? Activity can cause a child's blood sugars to drop like a stone. We know children who come home from a day sitting around at school with a blood sugar of 240 mg/dl (13.3 mmol), play actively for 30 to 45 minutes, and end up with a blood sugar reading of 80 mg/dl (4.4 mmol). This happens because it's not possible to take away injected insulin. In people who don't have diabetes, insulin levels fall during exercise. When anyone exercises with too much insulin on board, low blood sugars are often the result. (In Chapter 8, we discuss the hypoglycemic effect of exercise.)

If possible, your child should test her blood sugar whenever she's planning to exercise. If there's a chance she will go low during the activity, she can eat something first. She should also always have a source of fast-acting carbohydrate with her when she exercises, in case she begins to go low. Later in this chapter, helping your child learn to take these essential precautions is discussed.

Drinking Alcohol

If your kid drinks alcoholic beverages (even as little as 2 to 3 ounces), it can suppress glucose release from the liver, increasing her risk of hypoglycemia. When her blood sugar is low and she has been drinking, her liver loses its ability to pour glucose into the blood, leaving her without the safety net that could protect her from dangerously low blood sugar.

It may be hard to discuss this topic with your child, since she's unlikely to talk about it openly with you, but you should try, if you even suspect she might be drinking. Try not to be judgmental, if you can, and just share the facts with her, or ask her diabetes healthcare provider to raise the issue.

Drinking is risky business for any kid; having diabetes multiplies the risk. Your child needs to know that if she's planning to drink, she should eat something first. That way she won't be depending on the glucose reserves in her liver to protect her from hypoglycemia. Also, hypoglycemia can easily be mistaken for drunken behavior. Her friends should know about her diabetes, and she should have some form of diabetes identification on her. Hopefully, she will never drink to excess—it's just too much of a risk with diabetes—but if she does, these precautions will help protect her from a bad outcome.

Menstrual Cycle

Some young women tell us that their insulin requirements go down dramatically each time their periods begin and that they often need more insulin for a few days before periods start. Shifting hormone levels cause this pattern. If your daughter has increased her insulin doses to deal with rising blood sugars before her period begins, she may become hypoglycemic as her insulin needs go back down after the flow starts. If your daughter tends to have these fluctuations, she should keep close track of the pattern for a while so she can figure out how to raise and lower her insulin doses at the earliest possible moment and avoid these extremes.

Treating Hypoglycemia

No matter how hard you try, you can't always prevent low blood sugars, so both you and your child need to know how to handle them. Depending on your child's age and circumstances, you may not be there when they happen, and your child or another responsible person will have to manage the situation. Adults who spend a significant amount of time with your child (teachers, coaches, grandparents, friend's parents, youth-group leaders) should know what to do if your child has low blood sugar while he is with them.

Treat immediately. If you test and find your child's blood sugar is low, or if you can't test but you suspect she's low based on how she feels or how she's acting, get her something to eat or drink right away. All too often children ignore the early warning signs of low blood sugar. They tell themselves they can hold out another 10, 30, or even 60 minutes.

Kids generally hate to admit that they are low (it's embarrassing). They also hate to interrupt what they are doing. Unfortunately, delaying treatment can only lead to more severe low blood sugar.

Plan ahead. Have glucose tablets or another appropriate carbohydrate in your pocket or purse, in your car, or anywhere else you may need them. And encourage her to do the same. This seems to work best if it's the child's responsibility from the youngest possible age (with Mom and Dad also carrying or stashing backup supplies). Even very young kids can carry snack bags or have supplies in a book bag or backpack. However, as the story we told about Lindy at the beginning of the chapter suggests, this doesn't always work, especially with youngsters who are reluctant to reveal their diabetes to others. In fact, one of the most common frustrations we hear from parents of kids with diabetes is that their child will not carry food to prevent and treat low blood sugars. Sometimes this changes when the child has a scary or unpleasant experience, as Lindy did. We all learn best from our own experience.

Remember all the suggestions we made in Chapter 5, about helping your child learn to manage her own diabetes? She has effective veto power, so pushing her will not work, as you know all too well. The key is working with her to learn what would motivate her to carry the needed supplies. Make it clear to her from the outset that any suggestion you offer is off the table if she doesn't like it. That way she might not block you out, and you might get somewhere in your efforts to help her learn how to stay safe.

Specific Treatments for Hypoglycemia

Mild hypoglycemia. Mild, and even some moderate, hypoglycemia can be treated with 10 to 15 grams of fast-acting carbohydrate. Some examples are

- 2 or 3 glucose tablets (5 grams each)
- 1/3 to 1/2 of 30-gram tube of glucose gel
- 1/3 to 1/2 of a small tube of cake frosting
- 3 to 4 ounces of orange juice
- 4 to 6 ounces of regular soda
- 1/4 to 1/3 cup of raisins
- 5 Lifesavers candies

- 1 cup of milk
- Any high-carbohydrate, low-fat food that your child likes

If you're tempted to treat with much more food than these amounts, don't do it—at least initially. Giving more does not speed up recovery, and it may send blood sugar shooting way too high. Remember, high-fat sweets like chocolate and ice cream are not good treatment choices for most kids because the fat can slow down absorption of the sugar they contain.

Repeat the treatment in 15 to 30 minutes if your child's low blood sugar symptoms continue or if her blood sugar level is still below 60 mg/dl (3.3 mmol). The amount of food that will work best for your child depends on her body size and on exactly how low her blood sugar was to begin with. The smaller the body, the more rise in blood sugar that's produced by a given amount of carbohydrate. If you find that your child's blood sugars are consistently bouncing too high after treating low blood sugar, you might try cutting the size of the carbohydrate portion you're using.

If the next meal or snack is more than an hour away, you need to follow up the initial treatment of any low blood sugar with an additional carbohydrate snack that also provides fat. The easily absorbed carbohydrates that bring blood sugar up quickly don't last for very long—probably not more than an hour. That's why a more substantial and slowly digested snack is needed. Crackers and cheese, a peanut butter sandwich (whole, half, or quarter, depending on the child's size and how much longer until the next meal or snack), or a similar snack will protect your child from a recurrence of the low blood sugar.

Moderate hypoglycemia. Moderate hypoglycemia usually can be treated in the same way as mild low blood sugar, though it may take more than one treatment, and it may take longer to fully recover. The stronger the symptoms—confusion, clumsiness, slurred speech, headache, and so on—the slower the recovery. A child may feel perfectly fine within a few minutes after treating a very mild reaction, but it may take 30 to 45 minutes to feel totally normal again following a moderate reaction, so many people overtreat their low blood sugars. If you're feeling shaky, confused, ravenously hungry, and anxious, with your heart beating rapidly, you just want those feelings to go away! People tend to eat and drink until the symptoms are gone. It's hard to remember that it's the first 15 or 30 grams of carbohydrate that do the trick. One of our patients described his treatment for those lows like this: "I just empty out the refrigerator until I feel better. Last time it was about a quart of orange juice, two or three slices of bread, and half of a Snickers bar. My next blood sugar was almost 400 (22 mmol)."

Overtreating is more likely in children and adults who have had bad hypoglycemic episodes in the past. Kids may want to get back immediately to whatever they were doing before it happened and may have a hard time eating only the amount of food they need to get their blood sugar level back to normal. And parents can feel so panicked by their child's hypoglycemia that they tend to treat it too aggressively in hopes that the child will feel better that much sooner.

Risks of overtreating lows. It's natural to try to treat your child's hypoglycemia aggressively until she feels better. Unfortunately, if you give in to this temptation, her blood sugar is probably going to end up sky high. You might be able to curb this tendency if you use commercially prepared glucose tablets and gels to treat the hypoglycemia. These products are premeasured and not overly yummy, so you are less likely to overuse them. If your child simply can't stand these products, you might try preparing a low blood sugar first-aid package. It should contain just enough food (15 to 30 grams of carbohydrate) to rescue her from most low-blood-sugar emergencies.

Finally, you might use the approach (and try to teach it to your child) one of our patients came up with. She made up a little mantra that she repeated to herself as she waited for the food she had eaten to bring her blood sugar back up. It went something like this: "Relax, you'll be fine. You can wait a little longer. You'll be fine." The key, she said, was to keep the message reassuring and simple. Keep reminding yourself that you are doing the right thing and that everything will be all right. It may be hard to believe at that moment, but it's true. Try your best to stay calm and confident.

Severe hypoglycemia. When your child is severely hypoglycemic, by definition she cannot treat herself. She can't even ask for help, so it is essential that you or anyone else your child might be with at the time knows what to do. Everyone should know not to put anything in her mouth unless she is sitting up and able to swallow. We have seen tragic consequences when a family member tried to pour something sweet into the mouth of a semiconscious youngster. Usually, even with severe hypoglycemia, a person can be coaxed into taking something sweet. Stick with small sips of liquid, or try bits of honey, frosting, or glucose gel placed or rubbed between the cheek and gum. Avoid anything that needs chewing, because the coordination will not be there to do it and the child could choke. If you can't coax the child into cooperating, don't force anything into her mouth. Immediately inject glucagon or, if none is available, call 911.

Glucagon Emergency Kit

Glucagon is a natural counterregulatory hormone available by prescription in a glucagon emergency kit. The kit contains dry crystals of glucagon and a syringe full of liquid. When it is mixed and injected, it will cause your child's liver to release glucose into her bloodstream, raising her blood sugar level. Glucagon is the best treatment for severe hypoglycemia because it can be used immediately—no waiting for a paramedic to arrive, no wild ride to the emergency room—so the child spends less time at a dangerously low blood sugar level, and the whole family spends less time in a state of panic.

Every family dealing with diabetes should have glucagon on hand. If your physician hasn't already suggested it, we recommend that you ask for a prescription at your next appointment. And if your child has a history of severe hypoglycemia, don't wait even that long. Call now. You and other family members need to know when and how to administer it; your diabetes educator or other healthcare provider can show you. It is a safe drug, so you can't give too much. (Infants and toddlers typically receive half of the dose in the kit.)

Stored in the refrigerator, glucagon is good for several years. Since you probably won't need it often, occasionally check the expiration date and replace it before it expires. You are likely to be really anxious if you need to use the glucagon, so it helps to review the instructions periodically to stay comfortable with the process. Anyone who might need to give glucagon should do the same. (*See Table 7.2 for guidelines for using glucagon.*)

Medical Alert Identification

Medical alert identification can be a lifesaver. When your child is away from home, a medical I.D. bracelet, necklace, or wallet card will let

TABLE 7.2 Guidelines for Using Glucagon

- It's almost impossible to make a mistake giving glucagon. Inject in any site. Give the whole vial (or half of it for infants and toddlers).

- Make sure the person administering the glucagon knows to call for emergency assistance if the child doesn't respond to treatment within 15 to 30 minutes.

- Your child's stomach is likely to be upset after receiving glucagon; she may vomit. Turn her on her side after giving the shot. This will help prevent choking if she does vomit.

- As soon as your child is alert and able to swallow, offer her something light, such as soda or crackers. She must eat to replace the glucose stores that the glucagon has just released.

- As soon as your child is able to hold down food, have her eat something more substantial that contains protein and fat, such as a sandwich or some milk.

- If nausea or vomiting continues, contact your healthcare provider.

anyone coming to her aid in an emergency know that she has diabetes and takes insulin. Unfortunately, many kids resist wearing anything that announces that they have diabetes. If your child is one of them, be sure to offer her all of the choices available (necklace, bracelet, wallet card). Necklaces and bracelets are available in different metals and designs, so she should able to find an acceptable one.

One teenager we know, Sam, had several bad episodes of low blood sugar, but he refused to wear any of the commercial medical alert products, which drove his parents crazy. One day when he and his dad came to the diabetes clinic, a counselor found out that Sam was a talented artist and his father a skilled metal worker. The counselor suggested that Sam design a medical alert necklace he would be willing to wear and have his dad make it for him. They both loved the idea, and at an appointment several months later, Sam was proudly wearing the most awesome medical alert necklace we've ever seen.

Special Problems in Treating Hypoglycemia

Rebound Hyperglycemia

Although glucagon, the counterregulatory hormone, can raise your child's blood sugar level and protect her from becoming severely hypoglycemic, it can also backfire. If her body jumps in with its own protection before (or while) you or your youngster is treating it, the body gets a double whammy: all the glucose from the food plus all the glucose released by the glucagon. The result can be a stratospheric blood sugar level a few hours later.

If your child didn't have diabetes and her pancreas functioned normally, her body would simply put out some extra insulin to balance the effects of the glucagon and her blood sugar would remain normal. But because the pancreas doesn't function normally in diabetes, rebound high blood sugar can occur. What's worse, it can set up a roller coaster ride of more insulin to correct the rebound high, more hypoglycemia, and even more rebound hyperglycemia. To prevent the body from getting the real danger signals that trigger a further release of counter-regulatory hormones, it's important to catch and treat the hypoglycemia early, while it is still mild, whenever possible. This can also help to avoid those "clean out the refrigerator" treatment binges.

It's helpful to change insulin doses very conservatively and methodically after a bad hypoglycemic episode. If you can bring those rebound highs down slowly without overcorrecting and causing another low, you've done a great job.

Nighttime Hypoglycemia

Severe low blood sugar reactions happen most often at night. There are several reasons for this. First, most people have their lowest insulin needs of the day (often 20 to 30 percent lower than at other times) at 2 to 3 A.M.—the very time that NPH or Lente insulin taken with the evening meal is having its strongest effect. Also, a person is less likely to notice symptoms of hypoglycemia during sleep, so the blood sugar gets worse because it isn't treated.

To avoid nighttime hypoglycemia, always test your child's blood before she goes to bed. If the reading is low (usually less than 120 mg/dl [7 mmol], but check with your team), you may want to alter the bedtime snack to provide better protection against a nighttime low. This is especially important if she was very active during the day. Just giving more starch or sugar before bed will not necessarily provide protection when it's really needed, several hours later. You want something that will keep the blood sugar from falling in four or five hours. The things that seem to accomplish this best are fat and Lente carbohydrate, starches that are digested and released slowly. (*Refer to Chapter 6 for more information on bedtime snacks that protect against lows.*)

Getting the Job Done When Emotions Are Out of Sorts

You no doubt have noticed how low blood sugar changes your child's behavior. Sometimes it happens in subtle ways, maybe a little change in voice or speech pattern that only you are aware of; other times, it's more dramatic—your child becomes negative, irritable, or even verbally or physically abusive. And severe hypoglycemia may even cause her to act totally out of it, vague and disoriented, bumping into furniture, aimlessly picking things up and putting them down, or just sitting and staring into space. You may also notice emotional signs such as excitement, sadness, or rapid mood swings.

In any of these states, it can be difficult and frustrating to get your child to do something about her low blood sugar. She may fight you or simply refuse to cooperate, so you have to be prepared to manage the situation. Learn to recognize the signs of low blood sugar. Have a plan and the means for setting things right again. And find a way to deal with your own feelings when this responsibility is thrust upon you. Try to resist the natural temptation to lash out or to walk away from the whole mess. One mother we know kept her cool in a unique way. She'd tell herself that the person she was dealing with was not her darling son at all, but his evil hypoglycemic twin, and that her son would reappear magically when this was over. She said this little mind game helped her not take his behavior personally.

Finally, learn to administer glucagon. We know it's frightening to give your child a shot when she is lying there unconscious. The temptation to call 911 may be overwhelming. But if you teach yourself to use glucagon, you can give your child the fastest treatment and avoid the trauma and expense of dealing with emergency and hospital staff.

Hypoglycemia is awful. We hope that what you've learned from this chapter will help you to reduce the frequency of low blood sugars, and to treat them faster and more effectively when they do occur.

THE BOTTOM LINE

1. Low blood sugar impairs physical and mental functioning. It can also be scary, embarrassing, and even hurt family relationships.
2. Low-blood-sugar symptoms vary from person to person and from day to day. You and your child need to recognize her own unique symptoms.
3. Risk for low blood sugar rises with near-normal control and is caused by too much insulin, too little food, or too much exercise. Low blood sugar can often be prevented with planning.
4. Even when you're careful, low blood sugar can still happen. That's why you and your child must always be prepared to treat lows.
5. The right treatment given immediately stops mild hypoglycemia from becoming more serious.
6. Treat mild and moderate hypoglycemia with 10 to 15 grams of fast-acting carbohydrate. If the next meal is more than an hour away, follow treatment with a substantial snack.
7. Every family needs to have glucagon on hand. If you don't already have it, ask for a prescription and learn how to use it.
8. Medical alert identification can save a life in the event of severe hypoglycemia. Find something your child is willing to wear or carry.

8

Managing Sports, Food, and Diabetes

arry was a really active kid. His parents said he'd been running circles around everybody ever since he first climbed out of his crib on his own at the age of 11 months. Now that he was in middle school, his whole life revolved around the changing calendar of school and after-school sports. Football was followed by soccer and baseball, and then came summer vacation, with camp and swim team.

Larry was 12 the summer his diabetes was diagnosed. The first thing he and his parents asked for was advice about how to manage a coming swim meet. Larry didn't win any ribbons at that meet, but the fact that he swam in two events only two weeks after learning he had diabetes was a big victory in itself.

Larry was not the first child in the family to develop diabetes. His 14-year-old cousin, Becky, had been diagnosed six years earlier, when she was eight. "I'm not going to turn into a couch potato like her," Larry declared. The girl hadn't always been so inactive, but in

Larry had been running circles around everybody ever since he first climbed out of his crib at the ripe old age of 11 months.

the early days of her diabetes, a number of fairly severe low blood sugar reactions had greatly affected her and her parents.

The first time, she passed out while riding her bike and sprained her wrist in the fall. A few weeks later she nearly fainted while playing soccer. The third episode, complete with a seizure, happened during the night following a long hike with her Brownie troop. Her parents decided that it would be easier and safer to keep her inactive than to have so many low blood sugars. That was when Becky started spending most of her free time watching TV—a lifestyle Larry had no desire to share.

Whether they are participating in organized sports (like Larry) or just engaging in normal play (like Becky did before her parents lowered the boom), most kids have varied levels of physical activity. Balancing the right amounts of food, activity, and insulin can be a huge challenge. But handling it well keeps diabetes from being a barrier to activity— whether it's play or organized sports. And diabetes shouldn't stand in the way of so basic a need. A recent study suggests kids with diabetes are more likely than their siblings who don't have diabetes to be physically active, especially during their spare time. That's good news.

Organized sports and other forms of active play are a great way for your child to develop skills, stay in shape, spend time with friends, build self-confidence, and have fun. Ideally, active play should be a part of every kid's life; having diabetes makes it even more valuable. However, it does require your child with diabetes (and you) to plan carefully so that hypoglycemia and other potential problems don't spoil the fun, like they did for Becky.

Benefits of Exercise

Since exercise has a dark side for kids with diabetes (primarily hypoglycemia risk), why should we take the trouble to make it possible? Exercise has important physical, emotional, and social benefits that outweigh the hassle, so it's worth it!

Physical Benefits

A fit body. Strength, endurance, coordination, balance: All of these are a direct result of being physically active. Whether it's riding a bike with friends or playing on the all-state basketball team, exercise helps your child have the strong, healthy, flexible body that nature intended. As children move into the preteen and teen years, when appearance becomes more of an issue, the fact that a fit body is also an attractive body is another big plus.

A stronger, healthier heart. Did you know that most people with diabetes eventually die of cardiovascular disease, rather than kidney, eye, or nerve disease? This is the reason that heart health is very important for our children. When your child exercises, his muscles work harder and grow stronger. You may not think about it this way, but the heart is a muscle, too. Vigorous exercise builds the heart's capacity to work harder without straining, just like lifting weights builds stronger biceps. Exercise also helps keep blood pressure and blood fat levels normal, other important factors in heart health.

Lower blood sugar. You've probably noticed that when your child plays actively for even a short period of time (30 minutes or so), his blood sugar drops dramatically. Many kids come home after sitting all day at school with a blood sugar reading well into the 200s (+11 mmol), go outside to play for a while, and then come back in complaining of feeling low. Another blood sugar test may confirm that the blood sugar has dropped a lot (100 points [5.5 mmol] or even more). In fact, many parents help control blood sugar by sending a child out to play when sugars drift up. Be careful, however, that your child doesn't come to see exercise as a punishment for high blood sugars. Try instead to help your child see closer-to-normal blood sugar levels as a side effect of the play and sports he enjoys: a side effect you can sometimes use to your advantage.

The glucose-lowering effect of exercise is a good thing, but it can also be a challenge to stabilizing blood sugar control. This is especially true if exercise isn't consistent in time and amount (and few children play just as long and as hard at the same time every day). There are ways to manage this challenge successfully so your child can enjoy all the benefits of play and sports.

Weight control. Obesity is a growing problem among young people, and lack of exercise is a major cause. But not everyone is meant to be thin. Some kids are stocky by nature, others are average build, and a few are thin. Being active is especially helpful to kids who are already carrying around more body fat than is healthy or who have difficulty maintaining a healthy weight. Exercise helps normalize the appetite and keep it in tune with the body's real need for calories, so these kids can find and maintain the best weight for them without cutting back on the food they need for good health. Even quite heavy youngsters can stop or minimize weight gain through a combination of exercise and better food choices. This is also a more effective and responsible road to take than aggressive dieting, which is not recommended for kids who are still growing. A strategy like this allows kids to grow into the extra weight they're carrying, and it reduces the chances that they will get too hung up on how their bodies look or on dieting.

Reduced need for insulin. Since exercise lowers blood sugar, a child who exercises will require less insulin than if he wasn't active. Keeping insulin requirements as low as possible, consistent with good blood sugar control, is a good idea because it can mean a reduced risk of low blood sugars when the child isn't exercising and less likelihood of unwanted weight gain.

Emotional Benefits

Stress reduction. Kids need to blow off steam, let loose, get a little wild, and release the stresses of growing up. Exercise is a perfect answer to this need. You've probably had an experience like this: You're pulling your hair out because your child is bouncing off the walls and you send him out to play. Half an hour later he comes back in, happy and relaxed.

A better self-image. All kids need to feel good about themselves. A strong, healthy body that works as it should is a main source of those good feelings. Since your child has diabetes, he will almost certainly feel challenged in this area. That's why it's especially important that he be active and enjoy the positive feelings that come when his body looks and performs its best.

We know a pediatric endocrinologist named Dr. Raymonde Herskowitz-Dumont, who worked at the Joslin Diabetes Center in Boston, Massachusetts. Each summer she organized Outward Bound adventures for young people with diabetes. She took groups of kids 13 to 18 years old on sailing, canoeing, and scuba diving excursions. It was a powerful and challenging experience for the kids who attended, and they came away stronger and more confident not only in their diabetes management but also in every aspect of their lives. Not every child with diabetes can have this sort of opportunity, but participating in sports and active play can give them many of the same good feelings.

Social Benefits

Bonding and identifying with friends. Kids want to have fun with their friends, and being active together is one of the best ways. It breaks down barriers, strengthens connections, and allows children to communicate without words. It also teaches teamwork, sportsmanship, sharing, and healthy competition.

Strengthening family ties. Chasing your toddler around the backyard, hiking through the woods with your seven-year-old, playing a game of pickup basketball with your 11-year-old, or jogging a couple of miles with your teenager are all great ways to have fun and stay close. We'll talk a little later about how to make these family activities a regular part of your life.

The Risks of Exercise for Kids with Diabetes

While there are many exercise cautions for older people with diabetes, only a few of them really apply to children and teens. The risks for kids with diabetes include low blood sugar, very high blood sugar, and infections from injuries.

Low Blood Sugar

Exercise can lower your child's blood sugar too much if food and insulin are not properly managed to prevent it. Blood sugar can go low during play or exercise, immediately afterwards, or even many hours later. During and immediately after exercise, the activity can burn up all the available glucose, causing a low; later, it may drop even lower.

While your child is active, his liver is breaking down stored sugar (glycogen) to free up glucose to fuel his play. If your child is really active, he can use up all the glucose he has stored. For up to 24 hours after intense activity, his body will be trying to replace those fuel stores.

Any sugar that gets stored in the liver or muscles is taken from the bloodstream, which can create a risk for low blood sugar during the rest of the day following intense play or exercise. That's why it's especially important that your child eat all his scheduled meals and snacks in the hours after he's been active. He may also need extra food after he has played especially hard or long, even if he added snacks during the exercise.

Very High Blood Sugar

To make things even more confusing, another risk of exercise is high blood sugar. If your kid exercises strenuously, his blood sugar level can be driven up by the stress hormone adrenaline, which is released during exercise to help make more sugar available to the exercising muscles. A rise in blood sugar during exercise is more likely if your child's blood sugar was already high when he started and he had very little insulin on board.

Your child needs insulin to allow glucose to move from his bloodstream into his cells. With too little insulin, there is no way for sugar to get into the cells where it's needed. The cells, starved for fuel, signal the liver to make more glucose available. (The cells don't know there is already too much sugar in the bloodstream.) Sugar pours out of the liver but can't get into the cells because of the low insulin level. So the blood sugar notches up even higher. Finally, desperate because the cells still don't have any fuel, the body starts burning fat for energy. This provides energy, but it also produces toxic acids called ketones. As ketones build up in the bloodstream, your child can develop ketosis (along with the sky-high blood sugars). Not a good situation, to say the least. (It's similar to what happens when your child has a cold or the flu and his blood sugars get progressively more out of control.)

Checking for and clearing ketones. Any time your child's blood sugar is over about 250 mg/dl (14 mmol), he should check his urine for ketones. This is a good practice whether he is planning to exercise or not, but it's especially important if he is about to be active. Your diabetes healthcare provider will tell you the blood sugar level she considers critical.

If he has no ketones, it's probably safe for him to play. With a blood sugar that high, however, it's a good idea to take stock of where he is in the cycle of his insulin action. If his insulin is peaking or about to peak, he's probably fine, but if his insulin is running out, he needs to be careful. He might choose to take a couple of extra units of Humalog, Novolog, or regular insulin, or he might just check again for ketones in an hour or so. If the ketone test is positive (especially if the quantity is anything above trace), he has to clear the ketones with extra Humalog, Novolog, or regular insulin before the activity. Follow your doctor's guidelines for supplemental insulin doses, but be cautious about the dose if your child intends to keep exercising after the ketones are cleared. You don't want him to go too low.

Having ketones is rare for kids. This is fortunate because testing for ketones is universally despised by people who have diabetes—adults and children alike. We're not sure why—maybe it's because it involves messing with urine or because it could signal a medical emergency. If your child resists testings, try some of the questioning and problem-solving techniques we discuss in Chapter 5. You might admit that he hates the whole process, and you might sympathize with him. Point out how he would benefit from early ketone detection and treatment, and ask him how he wants to manage the situation. See if you can work out an approach together. Your doctor or diabetes educator may have additional suggestions.

Injuries and Risk of Infection

Kids with diabetes have the same risk for injuries that all active kids face, including the risk for blisters and foot injuries. However, they are more likely to have problems, such as infections, from any injuries that do occur. High blood sugars can interfere with normal healing, so they can slow recovery. This is another good reason to keep blood sugar as near normal as is safe and possible. (Good footwear makes injuries much less likely and is a must for active kids.)

Making Adjustments

When your child is physically active, you will need to adjust his food intake, insulin doses, or both to keep his blood sugars where you want them. Blood testing is the key to making these changes safely and effectively. Insulin and food needs during exercise are affected by many factors. To learn what works for your child in each unique situation, you must evaluate several factors: the time, length, and intensity of the exercise; your child's individual response to activity; his current blood sugar level; his insulin doses and timing; and the food that has been eaten or is planned. Armed with all this information, you and your child can greatly reduce his risk of exercise-related high and low blood sugars.

When Is He Playing?

A Saturday morning baseball game, a prelunch dance class, an after-school bike ride, and an evening soccer practice all require different approaches because insulin availability and meals are different for each time period (see "Guidelines for Insulin Adjustments" later in this chapter). You might deal with the risk of hypoglycemia during Saturday morning games by skipping or reducing your child's breakfast dose of Humalog, Novolog, or regular insulin or by adding more carbohydrate to his usual breakfast. The best approach for a prelunch gym class might be a larger midmorning snack; a little less morning Humalog, Novolog, or regular insulin; a little less morning NPH insulin (especially if the shot was more than four hours earlier); or some combination of these tactics.

A lot of kids run fairly high blood sugars at the end of the school day. If this is your child's pattern, after-school activities may not take any special adjustments. On the other hand, morning NPH insulin can also be working most actively then. The later in the afternoon an activity takes place and the closer to normal the blood sugar usually is at that time, the more likely it is that less morning NPH and/or a bigger afternoon snack will be needed to prevent low blood sugar. Evening games can often be dealt with in the same way as morning games: reduced insulin (usually Humalog, Novolog, or regular) in the premeal shot and/or more food with the pregame meal. Many active kids prefer insulin reductions, rather than food additions, because they don't like to play on a full stomach. Learning how to make these adjustments will take timely blood sugar testing and some trial-and-error practice runs.

How Hard Is He Playing?

Aerobic activities, like soccer or swimming, cause a more dramatic drop in blood sugar than anaerobic activities, like lifting weights. Running track or cross-country will probably push blood sugars down more rapidly than less strenuous activities like archery. Experience will tell you just how big a drop in blood sugar your child experiences with each type of exercise.

How Long Is He Playing?

If your child plays an entire basketball game, his blood sugar will drop faster and further than if he sits out most of the game on the bench. Of course, with team sports, you might not know before a game exactly how much your child will play. When the actual amount of time played is very different from what you had planned, it may call for extra testing as well as food (more play than you thought) or insulin (much less play) at the end of the game.

What Is His Blood Sugar?

Timely blood testing is essential to avoiding low blood sugar in active kids. Ideally, your child should test every time he's about to play. If that's impossible (or he's unwilling), figure out with him the time closest to the starting whistle when he can test. He should also have his meter handy, so he can check during the activity if he thinks he's low, although most kids resist testing during a game. If that's the case for your child, encourage him to eat something if he even suspects he is getting low. (*See specific suggestions below and in Chapter 7.*) It's better to risk being a little high than it is to let a serious low develop because of lack of treatment. If he is high, he might not perform to the best of his ability. But if he is really low, it could mean the end of the game— at least for him.

What Is His Individual Response to Activity?

Exercise affects everyone's blood sugar levels differently. Your child won't respond exactly the same every time, but you can learn a lot if you keep track of his levels. They will make more sense if you also record insulin doses and timing, the type of exercise, how long and hard he played, his food intake, and anything else that seems to affect them, such as illness. It's takes time, but it will really pay off.

How Much Less Insulin? How Much More Food?

After taking all those factors into account, decide whether you're going to change the food, the insulin, or both—and by exactly how much. Generally speaking, reducing insulin also reduces the need for extra food during exercise, but it seldom eliminates it entirely. Kids who don't have diabetes also eat and drink more when they're active.

Insulin and Exercise

You may notice some specific exercise-related changes in your child's response to insulin. For one thing, the same dose of insulin may lower his blood sugar more while he's exercising than it does when he's less active. For example, take a child whose blood sugar drops 50 points (2.8 mmol) for each extra unit of Humalog, Novolog, or regular insulin when he's going about his usual school day (*see the 1,800 and 1,500 Rules in Chapter 4*). He may find that each unit drops his sugar as much as 75 points (4.2 mmol) when he's running cross-country. The only way to figure out the specifics for your child is to review blood sugar, exercise, and insulin records together.

Exercise also increases circulation, so his insulin may start to work quicker than usual. The effect is strongest if he injects insulin into a part of his body that he is vigorously exercising (his serving arm if he's playing tennis, for instance).

Guidelines for Insulin Adjustments

In people who don't have diabetes, the body releases less insulin during exercise, which makes fuel more available to the muscles. Both the timing and the amount of the reduction are important. We can't be as precise in reducing insulin as the body is, but the following guidelines should help you make the necessary adjustments to your child's insulin for different activities.

- For light activity of any duration or moderate exercise that lasts an hour or less, it is probably easier to make any needed adjustments by adding food rather than reducing insulin.
- For moderate exercise lasting more than an hour and for any intense exercise, a combination of supplemental food and insulin reduction

will usually protect against low blood sugar better than supplemental food alone.

- Reduce the right insulin. In general, you reduce the insulin that is acting most strongly (peaking) during the time of the exercise. This will vary with the exact regimen your child is on. Keep in mind that insulin absorption can vary a good deal, changing its peak action time from person to person and from day to day. Use these generalizations about insulin action as a starting point:

  - Morning Humalog, Novolog, and regular peaks between breakfast and lunch.
  - Morning NPH or Lente generally peaks between lunch and dinner.
  - Evening Humalog, Novolog, and regular peak between dinner and bedtime.
  - Dinnertime NPH or Lente generally peaks between midnight and 3 A.M.
  - Bedtime NPH or Lente generally peaks around dawn.
  - Human Ultralente varies; it sometimes peaks slightly about 12 hours after it's given.
  - Lantus has no peak in most people, but in a small percentage of users, it acts somewhat like NPH.

- Humalog, Novolog, and regular insulin doses can be reduced or even eliminated entirely, depending on how long and hard the exercise will be.
- Background insulins (NPH, Lente, Ultralente, or Lantus) should never be completely eliminated. Start with a 10 to 20 percent reduction for exercise lasting more than 60 minutes. Adjust up or down on the basis of blood sugar results. Because of its very long period of action, Lantus should probably not be adjusted for exercise bouts unless they are so long or intense that they are likely to affect insulin needs for many hours.
- If exercise will continue all day (skiing, hiking, and other endurance activities), reduce the doses of all the insulins active during the day.
- For evening exercise, try moving predinner NPH or Lente to bedtime. It may not be necessary to reduce the predinner Humalog, Novolog, or regular as well, depending on the exact time, intensity, and duration of the activity.

■ Heavy exercise can reduce blood sugar for up to 24 hours after the activity is finished. If exercise is long or hard or takes place late in the day, you may also find it is necessary to reduce the insulin that acts after the exercise is done. For example, Todd played singles tennis all afternoon. To keep from going low while he was playing, he reduced his morning NPH by 30 percent. Then, to keep from bottoming out overnight, he also reduced his evening NPH by 20 percent.

The only way we know of to pin down the exact dose changes that will keep your child feeling and performing well is through blood testing: before, after, and often during exercise. We know the costs—both financial and personal—involved in frequent blood testing. But parents and kids also attest to the benefits, which is why we're so sold on the need for testing.

Guidelines for Food Adjustments

Even when insulin is adjusted downward for exercise, supplemental food may be needed, although the amount is likely to be less than if the insulin were not adjusted. And when insulin is not decreased for exercise, more substantial snacks are almost always needed. Sometimes parents don't give less insulin because they didn't know the child would be exercising, because the exercise is too short or light to call for it, or because they haven't gotten into making insulin adjustments yet. Here are some general guidelines for adjusting food, but the specifics will be unique for your child. You need to work them out through trial and error, on the basis of blood sugar test results.

■ About 15 grams of carbohydrate are needed to fuel each 30 minutes of moderate-level exercise in school-age children. The exact amount that is right for your child depends on body size (bigger bodies need more food for the same activity), the intensity of the exercise, and your child's individual response to activity.
■ If blood sugar is below 150 mg/dl (8.3 mmol) before exercise, your child should eat a snack first.
■ If blood sugar is 150 to 250 mg/dl (8.3 –14 mmol), it's probably safe for your child to exercise without more testing. However, testing is still a good idea if the activity will be intense or will last longer than

about 60 minutes, the insulin is peaking, or low blood sugar symptoms appear.

- If blood sugar levels are greater than 250 mg/dl (14 mmol), test for ketones before exercising. (*See "Very High Blood Sugar" earlier in this chapter for details.*)
- If exercise is long or hard, extra food may be needed in the hours after exercise to prevent low blood sugar. The body uses the extra food to replace stored glucose that was used up during the activity.
- Fluid replacement is vital to both performance and safety. Water is best, but sport drinks (with 10 percent or less carbohydrate) are fine, too. So are fruit juices diluted by half with water. Sport drinks or juice will provide at least some of the carbohydrate your child needs to protect against low blood sugar.

Recognizing and Preventing Lows during Exercise

Blood tests, together with food and insulin adjustments, will greatly reduce the number of exercise-related lows your child will have, but it won't eliminate them completely. Treatment for low blood sugars that occur during exercise is really no different from treatment at other times (guidelines are covered in Chapter 7). However, recognizing low blood sugars during exercise can be tricky.

Identifying reliable symptoms of low blood sugar caused by exercise. Some of the symptoms of hypoglycemia—sweating and increased pulse, for example—are also signs of an active workout, so you and your child might overlook them. You'll need to work with your child to identify symptoms you both can rely on. You might start by listing all the symptoms that he ever has when he is low. Put an "X" next to those that he also often has when he's active. Cross out the ones he rarely or never has when he is active. The symptoms marked with an "X" are the ones he should focus on as his most reliable early-warning signs of activity-related low blood sugar.

Identifying likely circumstances for low blood sugar caused by exercise. Develop a checklist of circumstances under which low blood sugar is most likely—things like, "Blood sugar was headed down before exercise"; "Didn't test blood sugar before exercise"; "Insulin is peaking"; "Long time since last meal or snack"; and any others you and he have discovered to be important. Then you can remind each other to be especially observant when those conditions apply.

Help your child learn a simple (but difficult to follow) rule: If you feel hypoglycemic while exercising, stop. If he can, he should test his blood. If he is low, he should eat or drink 10 to 15 grams of fast-acting carbohydrate—whatever he likes most and works best. Stopping, testing, and treating right away can be very difficult for a kid. But with your help, he can find the easiest ways to be safe. Go back to questioning and problem solving if necessary. What foods or drinks is he most willing to carry and consume? What will help remind him to take his supplies with him when he heads out to play? Does he have any other ideas to make stopping, testing, and treating easier?

Here's a summary of our suggestions for preventing exercise-related lows:

- Test blood sugar before, during, and after exercise.
- If exercise is very intense or will last longer than an hour, decrease the insulin acting during, and in some cases after, the exercise.
- If possible, time activity so that intense exercise does not occur while insulin is peaking.
- Avoid injecting near muscle groups that will be heavily exercised.
- Have snacks handy during all physical activity.
- Eat or drink extra carbohydrate at least every 30 minutes during activity that is intense or lasts a long time. Sport drinks or diluted fruit juices provide needed fluids as well as carbohydrate.
- Take extra carbohydrate at the first sign of hypoglycemia. Test first, if possible. If you can't test, take carbohydrate anyway.
- Eat more for up to 24 hours after exercise, depending on the intensity and duration of the activity and also on blood sugar levels.
- Learn individual blood sugar responses to exercise.

Exercise for Special Groups of Kids

The Very Young Child

Active play is good for everyone, right down to the very youngest kids. There are, however, some special concerns in managing the effects of activity in very young children with diabetes. For one thing, little ones tend to play in short, spontaneous bursts, which makes planning next to impossible. Instead of preventing blood sugar swings by changing food or insulin before exercise, you're often forced to cope with the lows that follow. In addition, very young children are less able to recognize that they're getting low and tell you about it. Because of this, parents and other adult caregivers need to be doubly watchful for signs of hypoglycemia.

For preschoolers, almost any activity can provide good exercise: walking around the block, splashing in the wading pool, romping at the park. Outings won't last long; even 20 minutes of active play at a stretch can give your child the exercise he needs—and increase his risk for low blood sugar. To make activity safe and enjoyable, you need to minimize that risk.

A young child is less likely to resist your efforts to monitor and manage his blood sugars. He'll probably kick up less of a fuss than an older child might when you test his blood before and after play or stop him midway to give him a snack. That's the upside. The downside, as we have noted, is that the young child probably can't yet recognize when he's getting too low. Even if he can tell when he's hypoglycemic, he may not be able to let you know about it. That's why it's especially important with little ones to have an early-warning system.

An early-warning system. Your early-warning system for low blood sugars has two players: you and your child. Start by learning to recognize subtle changes in your child's mood and behavior that signal dropping blood sugar. Then help your child learn to do the same as soon as he can. The most reliable signs may be unique to your child: an uncharacteristically grumpy mood, a sudden lack of coordination, a headache, a funny feeling, or even unexpected sleepiness. As we discussed before, symptoms can help, but they're never infallible. We hear all the time from parents who misread their child's behavior, assumed the kid was low (or not), and guessed wrong. Testing is the only way to know for sure.

To add your child's watchfulness to the early-warning system at the youngest age possible, help him identify how he feels when his blood sugar is too low. When you know he's low, ask him to tell you exactly how he feels. If he is unable to do this while he's low, talk about it as soon as he's feeling better. Keep it simple; he only needs one or two reliable symptoms to take care of himself. If he can't describe what he's feeling, try prompting him by asking if he's feeling shaky, headachy, sweaty, tired, or whatever other feeling you think might apply. It will take time before your child is able to recognize his lows, but it's never too early to begin helping him develop this essential skill. When both you and he are watching for the signs, your early-warning system is in place.

Food and insulin adjustments for activity. Very young kids' play is mainly spontaneous, so we usually make adjustments for activity with food rather than insulin. Because they're so small and their play is not very strenuous, they don't require very much carbohydrate. For example, our guideline earlier in this chapter suggests that most kids require 15 grams of carbohydrate for each 30 minutes of very active play. Preschoolers and toddlers often require much less, perhaps 5 to 10 grams for each 30 minutes of extra activity. Your child's past records of blood sugar, food, and activity can help you determine just how much he needs.

The More Serious Athlete: Organized Sports

Participating in organized sports can be a terrific experience for your child, helping him make new friends and feel good about himself. But all of the concerns we've already discussed, especially low blood sugars, need to be dealt with. Here are some tips that may help your very active youngster.

Bring the coach up to speed. For your child's enjoyment and safety, and for your peace of mind, your child's coach needs certain information. The bare essentials:

- Tell the coach what diabetes is.
- Explain that insulin injections, blood sugar testing, and extra food are necessary and will be required at times during play.
- Reassure the coach that your child can play safely and well, with certain precautions.
- Tell the coach how to handle any medical emergencies (small or large) that may occur.

For young children. If your child is young, his coach may sometimes have to help him with blood testing and treating lows. Some coaches are terrific: They deal with diabetes calmly and matter-of-factly and don't place any unnecessary limitations on the child. If your child's coach is such a person, you are blessed. If not, there's a lot you can do to help. First, you can educate the coach. Stick to the basic facts she needs to know. If you aren't quite sure what to say, check with your child's diabetes educator or other healthcare provider. He probably has material specifically designed to tell coaches, teachers, and others what they need to know. If information alone doesn't produce the desired result, try providing support as well. Be there—at least for a while—to handle the extra tasks and to offer guidance and reassurance. Most people learn best from experience, so if you help the coach be successful with your child and his diabetes, she will probably become much more confident and positive.

For older children. Depending on your child's age and level of maturity, he might want to talk to the coach himself. It doesn't really matter who provides the information, as long as the coach gets what's needed. If at all possible, follow your child's wishes concerning his role. In most cases, let your child tell his teammates. If he's not comfortable telling the whole team, make sure at least one buddy is in the know. This makes it more likely that your child will get timely help with low blood sugar even if the coach doesn't notice what's going on.

Try to help your child, his coach, and his teammates see your child's diabetes in the same way you do: something to take into account when he plays, but not a barrier to participation. With careful planning and good support, your kid can reach his athletic goals just as surely as if he didn't have diabetes. We know a young woman who has had diabetes since she was two years old; in high school she was the second-ranked long jumper in the United States in her age group. And most people are familiar with the experience of Olympic gold medalist Gary Hall, Jr. These are only two of many successful young competitors with diabetes.

Eating for competing. Food is fuel for competition. Fortunately, a healthy meal plan for a child who has diabetes—one rich in carbohydrates and low in fat with adequate amounts of protein—is the same one recommended for most athletes. For an active young person with diabetes, healthy eating helps fuel exercise at the same time that it helps maintain good blood sugar control. An ample intake of carbohydrates helps your child build and maintain adequate stores of glycogen in his muscles and liver, which is why eating well before, during, and after exercise is essential. Table 8.1 offers some suggestions for managing food for competitive sports.

Sports drinks. If your child wants a sports drink, try one with less than 10 percent carbohydrate. If the carbohydrate in a drink is too concentrated (above 12 percent, as in regular sodas and undiluted fruit juice), the body can't absorb it as quickly, resulting in nausea, diarrhea, bloating, and discomfort.

After the game. Good choices for carbohydrate replacement after a game include fresh fruit, low-fat crackers, muffins, granola or fig bars, oatmeal-raisin cookies, yogurt, soups, bread sticks, or pretzels. The extra food can be taken as an additional snack or added to planned meals or snacks.

TABLE 8.1 Food Game Plan

Pregame Meal

- Eat the meal one to three hours before starting time.
- Aim for a meal high in carbohydrates with some protein and a minimum of fat. "Lente carbohydrates" (oats, beans, lentils, cornstarch) increase the protection against lows for several hours after eating for some people.
- Good food choices include lean meat, fish, or poultry; potatoes without gravy or pasta with tomato sauce; vegetables, bread (no butter); salad with fat-free dressing; fruit; and skim milk.
- Drink plenty of water or other fluids before the game, including 3 to 4 cups of fluid with the pregame meal and more to drink before the event. This is especially important when it is hot or the event is long and intense.

Snacks

- If blood sugar is less than 150 mg/dl (8.3 mmol) before exercise, your child may need a snack of fresh fruit or fruit juice immediately before the game.
- For long and intense activity, your child may need a carbohydrate snack (approximately 15 grams of carbohydrate) during the game every 30 to 60 minutes. Sports drinks or diluted fruit juice may provide all or part of the needed carbohydrate.
- A postgame snack including carbohydrate may be helpful in warding off delayed exercise-induced hypoglycemia.

Adapted from Hornsby, WG, Jr (ed.): *The Fitness Book for People with Diabetes.* Alexandria, VA, American Diabetes Association, 1994.

Supplements. Some kids want to buy—or get their parents to buy— special meal supplements, power boosters, or vitamin and mineral formulas. These products are unnecessary unless your child is missing a particular nutrient, and they cost much more than foods that provide the same nutrients. Your child's success will be the result of his natural gifts and the work he puts into it, not the result of any supplements. If he wants to learn how he can boost his performance, attending a camp devoted to his sport or consulting with a registered dietitian who works with young athletes might be a better investment.

Kids who go overboard. Some kids, particularly in the preteen and teenage years, take exercise too far. They become too competitive and push themselves too hard. These children have an unhealthy commitment to exercise or athletic competition. When it is taken to an extreme, all that's good about active play can become a problem. Overly competitive kids can feel worse rather than better about themselves, lose friends instead of making them, and hurt their bodies instead of strengthening them. This intense focus on exercise may arise from an extreme need to win, a desire to be thin, parental pressure, or other factors.

Children who have diabetes certainly are not immune to these problems; in fact, they may be more susceptible to them, especially in the area of body weight concerns. For example, they may use excessive exercise to fight the tendency to gain weight if their insulin doses are not well regulated. If you think your child is going overboard with exercise, talk to him. If these conversations don't allay your fears, you might want to talk to his coaches or to his diabetes healthcare provider for further insight and advice.

Some adolescents try to control their weight by taking less insulin than they actually need. This behavior, which we call insulin purging, is an eating disorder unique to people who take insulin. It's a way to purge, or get rid of, calories consumed. (*See Chapter 9 for more about eating disorders.*)

The Inactive Child

Inactivity can be a temporary phase or a more persistent condition. Either way, it's a challenge to diabetes management and to overall health.

Your child's natural activity level. Some parents tell us their kids are classic couch potatoes. Their idea of exercise is channel surfing or hiking out to the kitchen for another snack. If your child seems to prefer being passive to playing actively, there are still things you can do to promote a healthier level of activity. But first, recognize that some kids will play less than others, no matter how much encouragement and support they receive. Einstein probably didn't spend his spare time mountain climbing. If your child is the contemplative sort, keep your expectations realistic. Individual or casual pursuits like riding a bike, in-line skating, or hiking might be more fun for him.

The right activity for your less active child. Let your imagination and his help you identify activities he might enjoy. Time and money place some limits on the available choices, but consider the possibilities. Walking the dog, dancing, biking (on the street or with a stationary bike at home or in a gym), aerobics, swimming, running, yard work, active housework, horseback riding, skating, skiing, rowing, all forms of team sports, bowling—the list goes on and on. Just make sure the activity is one he freely chooses. Use some of the problem-solving techniques we discuss in Chapter 5 to help your kid get moving and maintain his motivation.

Buying him some cool activity-related gear might do the trick, or taking him to games or lessons. Many parents walk, run, ride bikes, and play ball with their kids, and they have a great time. Pick an activity your kid is willing to do, and keep it simple at first. Starting off with a grueling hike is probably a bad idea.

Seasonal or Weekend Inactivity

Many kids tend to be active while the weather is good or they are playing on a team, but spend much less time playing in bad weather or during the off-season. Sometimes, weekdays are active and weekends are not. Such changes are almost always matched by changes in blood sugar control.

You have to adjust his regimen to restore balance when he switches between active and inactive phases. For example, when activity falls, he can decrease the amount he eats and/or increase the amount of insulin he takes. Eating less can be hard for some kids. It may take a while for their appetite to readjust to less activity, and meanwhile, they're hungry.

Although increasing insulin seems like an obvious answer, it might lead to unwanted weight gain unless handled carefully. There is really no perfect solution. The best approach during less active periods will probably involve some combination of reducing eating and increasing insulin.

Persistence and Flexibility

Unforeseen situations are a fact of life with diabetes, and being physically active adds another level of complexity to the mix. But meeting these challenges builds a degree of personal strength and diabetes know-how that is truly impressive. Needless to say, it takes persistence and flexibility.

Help for Every Active Kid with Diabetes

One wonderful source of information and motivation for any physically active person who has diabetes is the *Challenge*, the newsletter of the Diabetes Exercise and Sports Association (DESA). The DESA has branches all over the world, and the *Challenge* describes the adventures and accomplishments of its members. The stories are interesting, informative, and inspiring. For more information about DESA, write to

Diabetes Exercise and Sports Association (DESA)
P.O. Box 1935
Litchfield Park, AZ 85340
or call
Tel: 623-535-4595 or 1-800-898-4322
Fax: 623-535-4741
E-mail: www.diabetes-exercise.org

Your child doesn't have to back off from exercise, or even from athletic competition, because he has diabetes. But he does have more to think about and to plan and watch out for than his nondiabetic friends. And sometimes all this thinking and planning doesn't work, and he ends up with low blood sugar or some other crisis anyway.

A friend of ours who's had diabetes for more than 20 years tells a story about an experience he had at college just after he was diagnosed. He was walking across campus after an intense racquetball match when he realized that he had no idea where he was. He was sure this made no sense, since he'd been in the same spot many times before. Then it struck him that he must be having his first episode of low blood sugar.

He was desperate for something to eat or drink, but he didn't have any money with him. He approached a woman sitting on a nearby bench drinking a soda and tried to explain what was going on. Unfortunately, the sounds that came out of his mouth made no sense at all, not even to him. He grabbed the soda from the young woman and drained the can in a second. The woman leaped to her feet and went running across the quadrangle, screaming for help. He quickly fled before anyone came looking for him. His story reminds us of another thing you need to keep close at hand when you're dealing with diabetes: a sense of humor!

THE BOTTOM LINE

1. Exercise has important physical, emotional, and social benefits.
2. The major risks of exercise for kids with diabetes are low or high blood sugars. These problems can be prevented or minimized by a combination of blood testing and food and insulin adjustment.
3. Food and insulin adjustments are unique to your child and the situation. They are based on the current blood sugar, when and what he ate last, and when, how long, and how hard he will exercise.
4. An early-warning system for low blood sugars—in which you and your child learn to recognize when he might be low—enhances safety.
5. Diabetes need not be a barrier to competitive or strenuous activity. But it's much safer if the coach and one or more teammates are aware of the needs of a child with diabetes.
6. Encouraging the inactive child to be more active is just as important as helping the athletic child compete successfully.

9

I've got to be thin if I'm ever gonna make it as a dancer . . .

Recognizing Eating Disorders and Eating Problems

ennifer was a senior, majoring in dance at the local high school for the performing arts. She'd been very active in her own care from the time her diabetes was diagnosed at the age of eight, and her blood sugar control had usually been quite good. All of that fell apart around the beginning of her junior year. From that point on, her control steadily worsened.

By the middle of her senior year, her hemoglobin A1C levels were almost twice normal, reflecting an average blood sugar of about 350 mg/dl. Her weight dropped from 135 pounds to 116 pounds. During the first five months of her senior year, Jennifer ended up in the emergency room three times because of ketoacidosis. Needless to say, everyone was very concerned.

Jennifer's preoccupation with her weight captured her dietitian's attention, and he decided to have a long, serious talk with her. After a lot of encouragement, Jennifer finally admitted that she had been reducing her

Jennifer finally admitted that she had been reducing her insulin doses because it helped her keep her weight down.

insulin doses for months because it helped her keep her weight down. "I've got to be thin if I'm ever gonna make it as a dancer," she said. Her problems dated back to her junior year, when she had begun cutting back on her insulin doses occasionally so she could eat less. She discovered that when she cut her insulin way back, her blood sugars shot up and the weight just melted away.

Like Jennifer's family, Aaron's parents were beside themselves with frustration. The 12-year-old boy was never satisfied with the amount of food they provided, and he seemed obsessed with eating sweets and other junk food. Every afternoon when he came home from school, he tried to persuade his mother to give him a bigger snack. If he won, he greedily ate everything she gave him. If he didn't win, he'd sneak back into the kitchen later and get something anyway. Empty candy wrappers showed up in his dresser drawers, under his pillow, or in his wastebasket. His teacher even called home once to report that he was trading parts of his lunch for candy and cookies. Although Aaron's weight wasn't a problem, his blood sugars were far from good, and he and his parents were constantly fighting about how to get his eating under control.

Jennifer and Aaron both had eating problems related to their diabetes.

It's Hard to Eat Right

Why is eating well so difficult? Eating well is a challenge for many people, young and old alike, whether or not they have diabetes. Most of us, in fact, sometimes eat more than we should or eat things that aren't good for us. There are many reasons why we do this. For one thing, eating is pleasurable, and, for many of us, sweet and fatty foods deliver the most pleasure. Eating is also a social activity. Food is almost always included when people get together to have fun. We gather for breakfast, brunch, lunch, and dinner; for coffee and dessert; for pizza and beer; for holidays and birthdays; for weddings and funerals. Skipping the food often means missing out on a lot more than just calories.

Family traditions are also associated with food and eating. We want to eat the same dishes our parents and grandparents ate, and we want them prepared the way they always were. And as if all that wasn't enough of a challenge, more people are turning to highly advertised prepared foods and fast foods, many of which are high in fat, sugar, and salt.

Special challenges for kids with diabetes. Healthy eating can be doubly difficult for a young person, especially if she has diabetes. Your child wants to be just like her friends. She wants to be able to do what they do and to eat what they eat. Like them, she may have trouble controlling her weight, but when she overeats or chooses unwisely, she may suffer greater consequences than her friends do.

To be sure, not every child with diabetes struggles with eating right. For some, the challenges are no different than they are for kids who don't have diabetes. They occasionally overeat, eat too much junk food, or skip a meal or snack. But for others, the struggle is a truly desperate one, marked by bingeing and purging or severe restriction of caloric intake, disturbing and dangerous behaviors that indicate a clinical eating disorder.

Clinical Eating Disorders

The problem of eating disorders in people with diabetes has received quite a bit of attention in the past few years. There is some evidence that it may be more common in young people, causing serious consequences.

Anorexia nervosa and bulimia nervosa. Two particular disorders are most common. Anorexia nervosa involves severe self-imposed restriction in caloric intake, often combined with extreme levels of exercise. Bulimia nervosa involves binge eating followed by purging, usually in the form of vomiting or the use of diuretic medications or laxatives to get rid of the extra calories taken in during the binge. Diabetes offers another possible form of purging. By reducing or omitting insulin after binges, the child with diabetes can drive up the blood sugar, "purging" calories by rapidly washing them out of the body in the urine.

People with diabetes who have eating disorders are almost always in terrible metabolic control, and they often need to be hospitalized. Those with bulimia usually have chronically high blood sugars, and they may end up in the emergency room with ketoacidosis from omitting insulin. Those with clinical or subclinical anorexia, on the other hand, have low blood sugar levels pretty frequently, and they may need to be hospitalized for recurrent and severe bouts of hypoglycemia. Every aspect of the diabetes regimen becomes problematic for people with eating disorders: managing food, blood sugar testing, taking insulin on schedule, maintaining blood sugar control, and coordinating exercise with their treatment regimen.

Too much of a good thing. We know one young woman who became convinced of the value of tight control shortly after her diabetes was diagnosed. Unfortunately, she carried it too far, restricting herself to 1,100 calories a day. She tested her blood often, and her average reading was around 60 mg/dl (3.3 mmol). She went for almost two years with A1C levels below the lower limit of normal and often had low blood sugars. More than once, she required emergency medical attention to bring her back from a severe episode. Her approach to diabetes care was dangerous, but she was so preoccupied by fears of gaining weight and developing complications that she found it impossible to ease up on her regimen.

Clearly, both anorexia and bulimia carry short-term risks, but studies also show that young people who have eating disorders and a history of poor metabolic control develop complications (particularly retinopathy and neuropathy) earlier and more frequently than people without these disorders. In addition, some researchers have found that even people with less serious forms of eating disorders have worse metabolic control and more complications than those who are clearly free of these problems. This means that any disordered eating behavior should be taken seriously and dealt with.

How to Recognize an Eating Disorder

Common pressures on eating. How can you tell if your child has an eating disorder? The first step is to understand what's normal, so you have a point of reference for judging behaviors that are troubling and need to be evaluated by a professional. It's common in our culture for even quite young kids to be worried about weight. They are exposed to many "thin is in" messages, especially in advertising, but these common concerns are not exactly "normal," particularly in prepubertal kids. The value put on thinness is almost inescapable in our society, and it can cause great stress and self-doubt for those who don't fit the Madison Avenue mold of what's attractive. Obsession with being thin is more common among young women than it is among young men, probably because of the much stronger link our society makes between a woman's appearance and her worth. As much as we might deplore this and worry about young women growing up in this climate, it's not something that we're likely to change or solve easily.

Does your child have an eating disorder? Given this environment, it's understandable to want to be slender and to be disappointed if we're not. It's also normal to exercise to manage weight and stay fit and to overeat occasionally (or even fairly often). It's also normal to eat prunes or use other approaches to manage occasional constipation.

It isn't normal—and may mean that she has an eating disorder—if she

- weighs less than 85 percent of the normal range for her height, body frame, and age.
- has an intense fear of gaining weight or being fat, even though she is already underweight.
- sees herself as fat when others say she is too thin.
- exercises far more than is necessary to stay fit.
- misses at least three consecutive menstrual cycles.
- denies the seriousness of her low body weight.
- binges (eats very large amounts of food at a single sitting) at least twice a week for three months or more.
- feels she can't stop eating or control what or how much she is eating.
- induces vomiting.
- uses laxatives, diuretics, or enemas to lose weight.

In the realm of diabetes, it's normal to adjust insulin doses to maintain good blood sugar control. It is not normal, and strongly suggests your child has an eating disorder, if she purposely takes less insulin than she needs with the conscious intent of managing her weight. Insulin manipulation is an especially troublesome form of eating-disordered behavior, unique to people with diabetes. It is frighteningly frequent. In fact, some researchers estimate that as many as 50 percent of all young women with diabetes frequently take less insulin than they need in an effort to control their weight. Eating disorders are about 10 times more common among women than among men. This probably reflects the intense pressure toward thinness that is placed on young women in our society.

Severely restricting eating, bingeing, purging, and manipulation of insulin doses can all have disastrous consequences, leading to acute emergencies and contributing to chronic complications. For many young people, however, the appeal of thinness is so great that it makes all the risks involved in an eating disorder seem acceptable.

Kids rarely acknowledge eating disorders. Kids almost never voluntarily admit that they have eating disorders; in fact, they usually go to great lengths to cover them up. People who have eating disorders hide what they are doing because they're terrified that someone might try to make them stop. And they're often deeply ashamed.

It can be hard to distinguish between a normal (and even positive) focus on food and fitness and the abnormal concerns and behavior that reflect an eating disorder. Pay close attention to your child's behavior to see whether you find any signs of a clinical eating disorder. If you do see such signs, first talk to your child to see if she is willing to confirm that there is a problem. If she acknowledges that she's struggling, that's a good sign. Take action right away to get her the professional help she needs. We know it's difficult for you to be sure whether your child has an eating disorder. And we know it's scary to admit that she might have one. In spite of these feelings, it's important to get help for your child if you even suspect it.

We have already discussed the negative impact of these disorders on diabetes management. But it is also true that these disorders can actually be life threatening. And any degree of eating disorder is associated with sadness, shame, self-doubt and anxiety—which are painful and damaging on their own. Talk to her diabetes healthcare provider and ask for a referral to a mental health professional who treats eating disorders and, hopefully, also knows something about diabetes. They should be able to evaluate your child's situation, using screening questionnaires and a clinical interview, and treat her if necessary.

Some Types of Treatment

If you live in an area where there is a large diabetes treatment center, your child may be able to participate in a diabetes clinic-based group treatment program for eating disorders. The successful programs of this type are generally conducted jointly by the medical and mental health staff associated with the clinic.

Some individual psychotherapies have been shown to have some measure of effectiveness. However, overall success rates are not high.

One form of psychotherapy, called cognitive-behavioral therapy (CBT), addresses the thoughts, feelings, and behaviors associated with emotional problems, including eating disorders. Young people undertaking CBT to deal with an eating disorder work to modify their extreme beliefs about weight and body shape. This process is called cognitive restructuring. Recently, some researchers have reported successful treatment of eating disorders using the class of antidepressant medications known as selective serotonin reuptake inhibitors (SSRIs). This group of drugs includes Prozac, Serzone, Paxil, and Zoloft.

Regardless of the type of treatment chosen, hospitalization is often necessary. Medical hospitalization is required if the young person is malnourished or suffers from a mineral imbalance, problems that are more common with anorexia than with bulimia. Psychiatric hospitalization may be required to normalize eating behavior and to treat any associated psychiatric problems, such as depression, especially if the young person is suicidal. There are a few residential treatment centers that provide both medical and psychiatric support exclusively to those suffering from eating disorders, and your local mental health professional should be able to refer you to one.

If Your Child Denies the Problem

If your child doesn't acknowledge that she has a problem, but you're still worried, talk to her diabetes care provider for further advice. In addition, let your child know the following things:

- You love her very much.
- You are concerned that she might have an eating disorder, and there are reasons for your concern.
- You are available to talk about the issue any time she wants to.
- You are going to talk to her healthcare provider about your concern. You can suggest that she might want to do the same, if she is ever worried herself. You might also encourage her to talk to any other adult she trusts: a relative, teacher, religious adviser, or coach.

Ways to Prevent Eating Disorders

Given how devastating an eating disorder can be, you're probably interested in anything you can do to prevent your child from developing one. While there are no guarantees, there are some things that can help, depending on your particular situation. Most kids aren't vulnerable to serious eating disorders. For those who are, their parents' approach to eating, weight, and diabetes care may make a difference. First, take a flexible, individualized approach to your child's diabetes management—the kind of approach we describe throughout this book. If you insist on rigid standards for eating and blood sugar control, a susceptible child may respond by bingeing or avoiding food. Moreover, if you push too hard for tight blood sugar control, she may gain weight. Then, if that disturbs her, she may begin skipping insulin in order to get her weight back down.

Take a closer look at your own eating. You may also need to examine your own attitudes toward eating and weight. If you make a big deal about it for yourself or for your child, it can add to the pressure she feels to be thin. Remember, not everyone is genetically programmed to have a model's lean and lanky look. There are many people who are stocky or heavy, even when eating and exercising reasonably. If you are comfortable with and accepting of your body, it will help her like her own body and to feel comfortable with the shape nature provided. A susceptible child may still have problems because of the prevailing culture or the remarks and biases of her peers, but body criticism can be particularly painful and damaging when it comes from parents.

Think about the example you provide as well. A recent study found that young women with diabetes who had eating disorders often had mothers who also had signs of eating disorders. Do you have a relaxed and healthy attitude toward your own eating? Do you value fitness rather than fixate on your weight? Do you either binge or diet? Parents with such issues risk transferring them to their kids. They need to get help themselves so they can help their children.

Less Serious Eating Problems

Almost everyone has problems with eating at one time or another. Occasionally eating too much, having difficulty limiting snacks, or struggling to stick to a regular schedule of meals and snacks are common issues, and much less serious than anorexia or bulimia. Temptation, habit, social pressure, and stress contribute to these problems. Your child probably feels all of these pressures at times. And when she does, she may stray from the healthy eating practices you worked out with her diabetes healthcare provider.

Different kids will stray to different degrees and in different ways. For some children, sticking with a meal plan is relatively easy. They don't seem to be that tempted by things that aren't on the plan. They're happy eating what's better for them, and they're not particularly drawn to the sweet and high-fat foods that can cause trouble if eaten in large quantities. They find ways to manage social situations like parties and sleepovers without feeling awkward or deprived. Unfortunately, these kids are in the minority.

Healthy eating is a struggle for most kids. The majority of kids with diabetes get hung up on some aspect of their nutrition at least occasionally. They overeat, gobble up things that weren't planned or adjusted for, or refuse to stick to a schedule. These are common problems, and all kids have them from time to time. Nevertheless, parents get justifiably upset when these behaviors sabotage blood sugar control. The key to dealing with and minimizing these problems is to follow the parent and child job descriptions (*see Chapter 1*). They will help you avoid making mealtimes a battleground.

You want your child to grow up feeling that eating is enjoyable and relaxed, not a source of criticism, shame, and stress. To accomplish this, you need to work with your child to make mealtimes good times. For example, in attempting to get the right foods on the table, try to accommodate her tastes to a reasonable degree. We're not suggesting you cater to her every whim, cooking special meals on a regular basis, which could make her demanding and manipulative. But we are suggesting that you include some of her preferred foods in the choices at every meal and not force her to eat anything she absolutely loathes. Avoid going to war over cleaning up a plate.

Your child's favorite foods. Once you get the right stuff on the table, it's the child's job to decide exactly what and how much to eat. Children won't always choose exactly what you'd prefer, but as we discussed earlier, you can usually deal with this by offering choices instead of ultimatums. Use the Diabetes Food Pyramid to make sure the necessary groups are being included. If the overall food plan is reasonable, but she chooses to eat the same thing over and over, this can actually contribute to better blood sugar control by eliminating food as a variable.

You can bet that by the third or fourth time a kid ate the same meal for dinner, his parents knew exactly the right insulin dose and timing!

It's more work. Having some of your child's favorite foods available at every meal probably means extra work for you. Some things may be easy to make along with the other food you are preparing. Others may be prepared in quantity and stored in the refrigerator or freezer. If she loves chicken, you could broil or bake enough at one time for four or five dinners. You might also be willing to make her a sandwich in place of part of a meal she doesn't like. Only you know how much of this is really possible in your situation. As your child gets older, she will be able to do an increasing amount of the work herself. This can begin very simply: She can bring the cereal and milk to the table when it's okay for her to substitute cereal for part of her meal. When she's older, she can boil the water for pasta, prepare her own sandwich, or heat her own vegetables.

Shouldn't kids just eat whatever they are served? For many parents, the hardest part of applying this approach is getting past the feeling that the child should eat whatever is put in front of her. For some, it's almost a moral issue. For others, it's just an extension of the way their parents handled food. Expecting a child to eat every food that's offered sounds good, but in practice, it is often a disaster, whether a child has diabetes or not. And when a child does have diabetes, the potential fall-out is even worse. A kid with diabetes is already dealing with more than her fair share of eating issues. What she really needs is less pressure and the opportunity to make choices. She's much more likely to make healthy eating choices now and later if she feels she has some control over the situation.

Think of your own goals, as well. You want your child to be healthy and happy and to learn how to take care of herself, unencumbered by major food hang-ups. You also want mealtimes to be peaceful family occasions, not food fights. You are much more likely to accomplish your goals if you let your child make as many choices as possible, choose from the foods that you provide, and eat what her appetite dictates. Keeping insulin and food in balance while taking this approach is a challenge, but the benefits to family relationships are significant. Only you can decide exactly what's possible at your home, but we encourage you to stretch a little in this regard. We know you'll like the results.

Some Tricks to Smooth the Road

Plan meals ahead of time. Planning ahead can make following the parent and child job descriptions much easier. Some planning should be done well before mealtime. For example, try talking with your child before you do your weekly shopping to get her input on the menu and the shopping list. This can help ensure that at least some things she wants will be on the table. Make this a regular part of your routine so you both know the drill. If your child doesn't seem thrilled by the prospect, don't push it. Wait for the time when she's looking for something that's not there and suggest that she put it on the shopping list.

Or if she's willing, take her with you to the grocery store. Be clear beforehand that you will have veto power over any purchases she might suggest, but that you will try to be flexible. Some parents swear by having an occasional special shopping trip with their child just to buy the things she needs for snacking, treating low blood sugars, and so on. You don't need to do this every week, of course. It's just a way to ease your child into the meal planning process.

Finally, planning also takes place on the day of the meal. To avoid last-minute glitches, check with your child to be sure that you're including things in the meal she wants to eat. That way, if she's unhappy with the menu, there's still time for one or both of you to make adjustments. Does all this sound like a lot of work? We won't deny that it is, but it's a lot less work and a lot more productive than making mealtimes into a battleground.

Do as I say, not as I do. Your food-related attitudes and behaviors greatly affect your child's eating habits. If you nibble, nosh, or live on junk food, your kid will be more likely to do the same. We know this puts extra pressure on you, and since you (probably) don't have diabetes, you might think that this is unfair, that it's all right for you to eat as much or as little as you please. Unfortunately, it's not that simple. It's hard to help a child develop good eating habits when your message is, "Do as I say, not as I do."

What should you do if your own eating patterns are not the best? One option is to keep eating as you do and acknowledge that you are not living up to the standards you want her to meet. This approach may come back to haunt you when you try to get her to do the right thing, but at least it's honest. The other option—and the one we have found to work best—is to accept the challenge to change your own behavior. Change is difficult, but your efforts could bring great rewards: better health for you and for your child as well as a closer relationship.

If you do choose to change your own eating behavior, do it sensibly and gradually. Going on a crash diet won't help, and it sends your child the wrong message. Try to follow the healthy eating guidelines in Chapter 3. A nutritionist could help if you are having problems getting started or if you need support.

Control the eating environment. Environmental control can be a big support in maintaining healthy eating habits. Most people find they are more likely to eat sensibly if they put on their plate only the amount of food they are planning to eat, and leave the rest on the stove. Some even pack it away in the refrigerator or freezer once the plates have been filled. We think this is a great idea, as long as you stay flexible and can provide more food if people want it. Also make sure that the amount you're portioning out is appropriate—remember, if a child is either hungry all the time or leaving a lot of food uneaten, the portions probably need adjusting. Traditional family-style eating, with a whole plateful of meat, a loaf of bread, a bowl of vegetables, and everything else on the table, can be a set-up for overeating. You and the kids may keep eating to "clean it up," not because you're really still hungry. Sitting down with only the food you intend to eat may be a good solution for some families, but it will be awkward or difficult for others. Still, it can help you keep track of exactly how much is eaten, and it keeps the business of portion control off the table. Give it a try. Another technique is keeping junk food out of the house or buying it in small quantities that are likely to be eaten at a single sitting. If it isn't there, it's hard to eat it!

Don't expect perfection. You'll also help to minimize your child's eating problems if you check out your expectations for her behavior. Perfection is no more a possibility when it comes to your kid's eating than it is in blood sugar control. Parents who expect perfection often find that their children become overwhelmed by the unrealistic standard and then just say, in effect, "To hell with it. I'm blowing it anyway; how much doesn't matter." But, of course, how much does matter. Or they may begin to hide what they're really doing from parents who they know would be upset by the truth.

The challenge in encouraging healthy food choices is to be both ambitious and realistic. Healthy eating and excellent blood sugar control are wonderful goals. But be flexible. There are many choices to be made as your child learns to take good care of her diabetes. Help her see that she still has plenty of choices, even though her diabetes limits them somewhat. Ask her questions about the food-related situations she finds hardest to manage, and then really listen to the answers. Ask her what makes these situations easier to manage. Find out if there's anything you can do to help. Help her learn how to control her own blood sugar. A flexible, accepting, problem-solving approach will make that far more likely than fruitlessly demanding perfect behavior.

Follow your job description. Get help if you notice signs of disturbed eating. Most important of all, love your child as she is, support her in becoming all she can be, and make sure you two stay on the same side of the fence.

THE BOTTOM LINE

1. Most people sometimes eat more than they should or eat things that aren't good for them. These behaviors run the gamut from garden-variety issues about food to full-blown clinical eating disorders.
2. Young people with diabetes, especially young women, are at higher risk for such problems.
3. Young people who have diabetes and a clinical eating disorder (anorexia nervosa or bulimia nervosa) almost always have terrible blood sugar control.
4. The symptoms of a serious eating problem include low body weight, fear of being fat, excessive exercise, abuse of laxatives, binge eating, self-induced vomiting, and taking much less insulin than is needed. If you notice any of these symptoms, it's vital to get help.
5. A mental health professional who treats eating disorders can evaluate the situation and provide treatment, if needed.
6. Parents can help prevent both common and more serious eating problems in susceptible children by successfully managing their own eating, confronting their own attitudes about food and weight, and following the parent and child job descriptions.

It seemed like I'd just finished feeding, diapering, and testing his blood, and there he was, crying for the next feeding.

10

Babies and Toddlers

Corey was only a little over two months old when his diabetes was discovered. As is often the case when babies and toddlers develop diabetes, he had become really sick before anyone realized something was wrong. He had to be admitted to the hospital because of DKA (diabetic ketoacidosis), a serious condition caused by lack of insulin. He was "limp as an old dishrag," according to his mother. The pediatrician and nurse were very sympathetic and willing to help, but since babies with diabetes were pretty rare in their small, agricultural town, the professionals didn't have much practical advice to offer about Corey's day-to-day care.

"You'll just have to do a lot of blood tests," the doctor informed them. "That's the only way we can figure this out. Test before and after every feeding, before you put him down to sleep, and anytime he's acting unusual."

Corey was their first child, so the young parents didn't know exactly what the doctor meant by "unusual" behavior. As a result,

What if a cry meant he was hypoglycemic instead of just wet or hungry?

there was a lot of testing going on, at least at first. What if a cry meant he was hypoglycemic instead of just wet or hungry? But the number of tests dropped off quickly once they realized the costs involved. They just couldn't afford to do the number of tests the doctor recommended. Their HMO provided one vial of test strips per month, which didn't even get them through the first week after they brought Corey home from the hospital. Once that vial was gone, every additional test costs 70 cents each.

They also hated the upheaval the tests caused. Corey's mom hated doing a blood test before feeding him because the baby got so upset. He'd always been an eager feeder and didn't tolerate a lot of dallying around once he decided he was hungry. The delay in his feeding and the further indignity of being stuck in the heel created a totally unacceptable situation in the baby's view. As his dad described it, he "went nuclear." Mom and baby were both a wreck by the time she sat down to nurse. All this stress seemed to be interfering with her milk supply, so she was skipping as many of the blood tests as she could. Corey was nursing every two to three hours on average, and with feedings so close together and so many things to do at each one, no one was getting any rest.

Blood sugar control was poor and was generating 12 to 15 wet diapers a day. More diapers, more expense, more stress. And the baby wasn't gaining any weight. No one knew for sure whether this was due to the disruption of Corey's feeding, to a problem with Mom's milk supply, or to the diabetes itself (because of poor blood sugar control).

After close to six weeks of this, Corey's pediatrician was feeling just about as overwhelmed as the parents. It took several heated phone conversations for the doctor to convince the HMO that the family needed to be seen right away by a pediatric team in the nearest large town.

Corey's story highlights several common issues among families with diabetic babies. Corey's mom and dad were feeling uncertain and overwhelmed, a universal reaction of parents whose infants develop diabetes. Caring for the baby was taking up nearly all of their waking hours. They worried about hypoglycemia constantly and wondered about the meaning of every cry, burp, and twitch. They were uncertain about whether he was getting enough food. Finally, they were emotionally and financially strapped.

The medical personnel in their town didn't have much experience with diabetes in babies. This is often true even in large cities, because there just aren't that many babies with diabetes. Most children develop diabetes at a later age, so even doctors who see a fair number of these older children may have very little hands-on experience with an infant. Certain aspects of care are unique to this age group, and parents have to learn them the hard way, by trial and error. But by the time they master the ins and outs of their baby's diabetes management, the child has grown into a new set of challenges.

Every family with a diabetic infant struggles with balancing the need to know the blood sugar level against the cost and discomfort of testing. Understandably, everyone absolutely hates to stick a baby. Yet the test results provide extremely important information, because the baby can't tell you if he's feeling sick or low.

Finally, the questions and concerns about Corey's feedings are also typical for the families of babies with diabetes. The milk feeding— whether it's breast milk or formula—is the sole source of nutrition for babies younger than five or six months of age. How it's managed is absolutely vital to the baby's overall health. But the details of how to keep the milk and the insulin in balance are neither easy nor obvious.

A daunting situation, to be sure. But there are some tips and techniques that can lighten the load.

Babies

First of all, rest assured that your baby with diabetes is going to grow and develop normally. Keeping blood sugars in reasonable control helps ensure this. Your doctor will track the baby's growth on a grid, similar to the ones shown in Figures 10.1 and 10.2. (Growth grids are explained in Chapter 2.) But here's a concern that applies to babies and toddlers especially: The length entered on the grid may not be correct, because babies squirm and don't like being stretched out on those measuring tables. And even when babies get big enough to stand, things might not get much better. If the pattern on the growth grid doesn't make sense to you, ask the doctor or nurse to measure again. If your baby is gaining steadily, has strength and energy, is nursing and eating contentedly, and doesn't seem particularly hungry or lethargic, that's pretty powerful evidence that he's doing fine.

There may be a short setback in development right around the time your baby's diabetes is discovered. This is generally true of babies with any kind of health problem. Once this blip is past, all of the developmental milestones of infancy—sitting up, walking, talking, and so on—should happen according to your baby's proper timetable.

BOYS: BIRTH TO 36 MONTHS
PHYSICAL GROWTH
NCHS PERCENTILES*

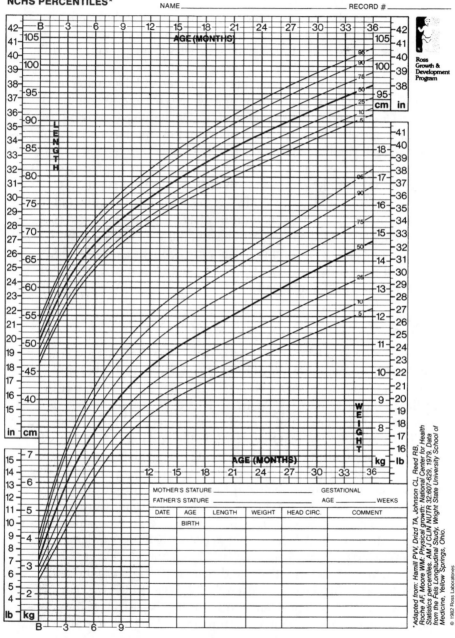

FIGURE 10.1 Growth Grid for Infant Boys

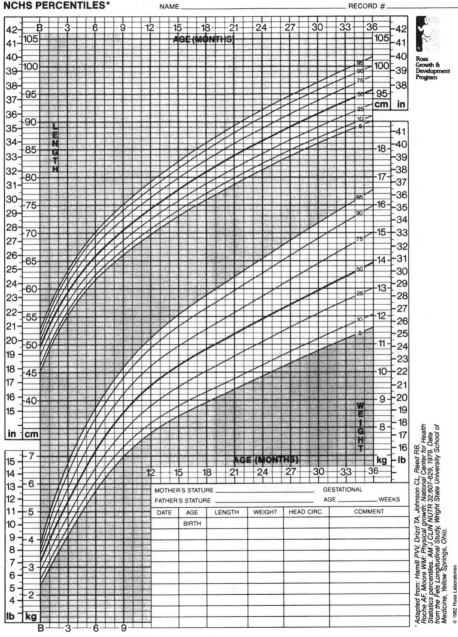

FIGURE 10.2 Growth Grid for Infant Girls

A baby with diabetes needs lots of love, care, closeness, and nurturing—just like every other baby. Some of the closeness will now be connected with diabetes care routines—in particular, shots and blood tests. Parents tell us there are tricks that help take some of the sting out of these tasks. Making the daily pokes with needles and lancets less stressful can do a lot to help everyone's frame of mind. And from a nutritional viewpoint, keeping everyone a bit calmer promotes better feeding.

Here are some words of advice from parents who've been there. Avoid sneak attacks to do shots and blood tests. Babies and older kids alike may get paranoid and start to flinch every time you pick them up for a cuddle. Instead, consider setting up a diabetes care station where you keep the supplies. Do all the shots and blood tests there while you're at home, at least until your child gets older and more accepting of the routine. Distract the baby at the critical moment or have someone else do it: Patting or squeezing another part of the body works well, as does offering a favorite toy. You may want to use plastic pipettes (some folks call them Barbie Basters) to transfer blood from heel or finger to the strip. This cuts down both on having to control a squirming baby and on wasting strips because of an ill-timed kick or lunge. When you're done, cuddle immediately and thoroughly. If the child has gotten teary or upset, cuddle until he's calm before trying to nurse or feed him, if at all possible.

Newer Meters Can Cut Discomfort and Hassle

Look for a meter that requires the smallest blood sample possible. Stay away from those that need a big, hanging drop. New meters use much less blood, and "alternate site" meters allow you to test on the arm instead of sensitive fingers. Most people don't feel any pain at all from them, so they're great for families with kids.

Be aware, however, that blood sugar levels don't change throughout the body at the same rate. When blood sugar is changing quickly, the change will show up sooner in fingers and toes than on the arm or leg. So, when using an alternate site meter, it's probably a good idea to test fingers or toes if you think the blood sugar is falling or rising quickly. But even fingertip tests with the Freestyle (Therasense) and the Ultra (Lifescan) are likely to be more comfortable because they take such small blood samples.

Testing technology is advancing very quickly along several fronts. Everyone is still anxiously awaiting noninvasive and minimally invasive testing, which would not require blood to be drawn. One promising new device that has been approved by the Food and Drug Administration is the GlucoWatch Biographer, by Cygnus. It is a noninvasive, watchlike device that has an automatic sensor to detect blood sugar levels. It can provide blood sugar readings for up to 12 hours at a time. In addition, an alarm sounds if blood sugar is too high or too low. However, the device is very sensitive to movement and perspiration, and some people develop irritation from it. Blood tests must still be done to calibrate it and to confirm the sensor's readings.

A Role for Urine Tests

Blood tests are the only way to confirm low blood sugar, and regular blood tests are vital to knowing your baby's pattern of control. But extra blood tests sometimes can be avoided by doing urine glucose tests on your baby. This can help cut both costs and tears, especially when your main concern is high blood sugar. Urine glucose testing doesn't give you a specific blood glucose number, but it does allow you to confirm high blood sugar. For example, if your baby is wetting more diapers than usual, leading you to think he's running high, you can often confirm it with a urine test. You may be able to do a urine catch at the time of a diaper change. If not, you can wring a few drops of urine out of a wet cloth diaper or diaper liner (most disposable diapers that "don't leak" contain silica gel, which makes it impossible to squeeze urine out of them). Not perfect, but a helpful bit of information gathered at a smaller cost—both financial and personal.

Don't forget that there is a time lag between actual blood sugar and a urine test result. If the urine you're testing was made some time before you do the urine test, the blood sugar may have had time to drop in the meantime. That time lag, which can be several hours or more, and other uncertainties are why we *never* adjust insulin on the basis of urine sugar.

Urine either from the diaper liner or from a urine catch done at changing time can be used to do urine ketone tests as well. Your doctor will tell you when these are needed—most likely anytime the baby is sick or has very high blood sugar.

Hypoglycemia in Infants

Low blood sugars are scary and potentially dangerous in infants. That's why most doctors set somewhat higher glucose targets for infants and very young children than for school-age and older kids. Keeping blood sugar a bit higher—say, making 100 mg/dl (5.6 mmol) the lowest acceptable blood sugar—gives you a bigger margin of error and is one of the most effective ways of protecting your baby against excess low blood sugars.

Another important prevention tactic is to avoid force-feeding. When parents force, it almost always leads to babies actually eating less. This is true both of milk (breast-feeding or formula) and solids, once they're started. Be alert to your baby's signs of hunger—for example, the type of cry that distinguishes hunger from a wet diaper or from general fussiness. Then offer breast, bottle, or solids in a calm, matter-of-fact fashion. If not forced, hungry babies will usually eat eagerly. However, if the baby takes much less than usual because he isn't particularly hungry, be on the alert for signs of dropping blood sugar in the hours after the feeding. Once blood sugar is on the way down, most babies nurse or eat willingly if you catch it early and calmly offer breast or bottle.

Insulin management in babies is tricky. They don't eat major meals the way we do, and their intake is variable and all but impossible to change. For these and other reasons, most doctors don't use any short- or rapid-acting insulin in babies and toddlers, unless they're wearing a pump. (Pumps use only rapid-acting insulin but can deliver it constantly in tiny amounts so there are no peaks—unless you program them in.) Two or three injections of intermediate- or long-acting insulin or one injection of Lantus (insulin glargine) will spread insulin out as evenly as possible through the day. This is well suited to the way babies graze, eating and drinking small amounts multiple times throughout the day. Not using short- or rapid-acting insulin means fewer strong insulin peaks and affords some protection against low blood sugars. Blood test results help you and the doctor keep the baby's insulin doses adjusted to his food intake and to the changing needs created by growth and development.

Insulin adjustments in babies need to be very small. That is one reason why pumps are gaining in popularity. Pumps can deliver as little as 1/10 unit of insulin accurately. The best you can do with a pen is a half unit, which is a lot of insulin in a tiny little body. Bigger dose adjustments may lead to radical changes in blood sugar. That's why it's not uncommon to dilute insulin for babies and toddlers to make it possible to give very small doses by syringe more accurately. If your doctor decides that dilution would be helpful, be sure that someone teaches you how to do the dilution and how to measure doses correctly for the specific dilution and syringe you're using. This is a very precise process and not one you should try to learn on your own.

Even with careful insulin management, hassle-free eating, and modified blood sugar goals, babies will still become hypoglycemic at times. And, of course, they can't tell you what's going on. It helps to become familiar with your baby's particular symptoms of falling blood sugar. There are a lot of possibilities. Your baby might have a particular cry, become pale or cranky, start to sweat or tremble, or develop a bluish tinge to fingers or lips. Symptoms are your early warning system. They are your sign to test. If you can't test, treat anyway. It's safer than waiting to see what happens. Brain development requires a constant supply of glucose, which is why preventing low blood sugars in infants, whose brains are still developing, is a high priority. Low blood sugars must also be treated as quickly as possible to ensure that the blood sugar doesn't stay low for long.

To treat low blood sugar in an infant, offer a drink with easily absorbed sugar. Apple juice seems to be preferred, but anything that works well for your baby is fine. It probably won't take a lot. Carbohydrate goes much farther in a small body than it does in a larger one—a mere 5 grams (the amount in about 1 ounce of juice or 2 ounces of sugar-sweetened Kool-Aid) usually does the trick for a baby or toddler. Once the blood sugar is back up, follow the sweet drink with formula or breast milk to keep it there. In older babies who are taking solids, cereal or bread with egg or another source of fat could be offered as a follow-up instead of milk.

Glucagon is needed if the baby won't eat or if the treatment doesn't seem to be working (*see Chapter 7*). Every home with a child who has diabetes needs to have glucagon on hand.

Feeding Infants

The milk feeding. From birth until about four to six months of age, milk is the baby's only source of nutrition. Either breast-feeding or bottle-feeding with formula will produce a healthy baby. If you're breast-feeding when your baby develops diabetes, you'll need to weigh the advantages of it against the reassurance a bottle provides in seeing how much the baby has consumed. If you're trying to make this decision right now, keep this in mind: Trying to wean a baby from breast to bottle when you're also dealing with the unfamiliar demands of diabetes care won't make things any easier. If you do decide to continue breast-feeding, be aware of the mother's stress level, rest, fluid intake, and nutrition, any of which can interfere with the milk supply. If the baby is admitted to the hospital at diagnosis, this decision may be taken out of your hands and the baby placed on formula to simplify things for the hospital staff. However, if you're determined to breast-feed, talk to the staff about your wishes. Breast milk can be pumped for any feedings when Mom won't be there to provide the real thing. Pumping will help keep your milk supply strong, even if not all the milk is used.

Starting solids. A baby first needs solid foods at around four to six months of age. His nutritional needs are changing and his development demands it. He's becoming able to coordinate tongue and jaws in such a way that swallowing solids becomes possible. The strong gag reflex of infancy is decreasing. He is able to sit up without support. The stage is set to move on to his next phase, eating semisolid and solid foods. Giving solids at younger ages doesn't have any nutritional benefits.

When solids are first started, practicing the skill of eating is actually more important than the foods themselves. Milk or formula should still be the major source of nutrition. Solids shouldn't displace milk until a child is well established on a variety of table foods. This generally happens somewhere around one year of age, or a bit older.

The first nutritional need to be met by solids is that for iron. Milk is not a great source of iron and the extra supply he was born with is starting to run out. So the preferred first solid food is often baby cereal fortified with iron. It should be given by spoon in a semisolid consistency. Each 2-tablespoon serving prepared with milk provides about 5 grams of carbohydrate. At about six to eight months, fruits, fruit juices, vegetables, and "finger breads" (teething biscuits, arrowroot cookies, etc.) can be added one at a time. Two-tablespoon servings of fruit provide about 4 to 5 grams of carbohydrate, as does each ounce of fruit juice. There is no real need to include protein foods this early, since the baby will still be getting adequate protein from the milk feeding. Meats and eggs can be added at around 7 to 10 months, when the baby begins to graduate to table foods.

Sometimes, it's tricky to figure out how much a baby (or toddler) has actually eaten. Do you count what's smeared on the high chair? No, but how do you know how much got past the lips versus how much ended up as wallpaper? We don't have a clear answer. Parents of the youngest children with diabetes seem to favor retrieving food from faces, trays, and bowls and reoffering it for as long as the baby is still eating willingly. An inexact science at best. But we can tell you that smearing, spitting, and throwing generally escalate after the child's had about enough. Try to take stock of how much was eaten before the pablum hit the fan.

There is no reason to give babies artificially sweetened drinks. They get plenty of sweetness from fruits and fruit juices. Some families of diabetic infants use sugar-sweetened Kool-Aid or punch to treat low blood sugar, which is fine. But using artificially sweetened drinks when the baby is just thirsty may unnecessarily encourage a preference for sweets. Plain old water is probably the best beverage for babies, beyond the milk feeding and the small amount of fruit juice needed for vitamin C and the occasional low blood sugar.

As the baby's meals become more substantial, moving carbohydrate around in the day can help keep insulin demand in balance with insulin availability. For example, if high blood sugars are a problem at midmorning, some fruit, fruit juice, or starch could be moved from breakfast or the morning snack to noon or later, when morning NPH, Lente, or Ultralente may be having a stronger effect. Vegetables or meat could be given in their place in the morning feeding. These choices would still satisfy the baby's hunger but have less effect on blood sugar. Distributing carbohydrate foods throughout the day, instead of grouping them at certain feedings, can help with glucose control and may help delay the need for adding rapid- or short-acting insulin to the treatment plan.

Toddlers

Perhaps it's true that dealing with a toddler is nature's way of preparing us for teenagers, as some have suggested. There are certainly similarities between the two. Toddlers are proving to themselves and to you that they are separate people. Teenagers are trying to prove the same thing to the whole world. Resisting you is an excellent way to prove that separateness, and so a toddler's favorite word is "No!" He very much wants to explore and be independent, but at times, it scares him to death. Your job at this stage is to let him explore, help him be successful as he tries new things, and yet set clear limits. Without limits, the two-year-old and the teen will push and push until you're forced to step in. Setting and maintaining reasonable limits is also important in feeding the toddler.

Toddlers Do Best with Choices

This is the age of self-feeding, so make food easy for him to eat on his own. Give him his food already cut into bite-size pieces. Leave the dressing off his salad so he can eat it with his fingers. Stay away from things that are too dry or tough for him to manage easily on his own. According to the parent and child job descriptions discussed in Chapter 1, you get the right stuff in front of the child and decide when, where, and how the meal or snack will take place. The child decides how much he will eat of what you offer. Trying to force a toddler to eat is like poking a short stick into a pile of sleeping rattlesnakes. You will not be happy with the result!

Avoid fighting and scolding during meals at all costs. This will have a negative effect on your child's eating in both the short and the long term. The best way to keep the peace is to have plenty of acceptable choices available: choices that you know your toddler enjoys and that meet the current demands of diabetes control. When your main concern is getting enough food into the child to cover insulin, offer different choices or bigger portions of things you know your child enjoys. When the toddler has eaten all the planned meal and is yelling for more, offer choices with less blood sugar impact, like proteins, fats, and low-carbohydrate vegetables.

This is the age when children learn how to manage silverware, but keep in mind that they'll be total klutzes at first. Show your child how it's done by doing it yourself. Praise him for whatever he's able to manage reasonably well. He'll pick it up eventually by watching you and practicing, so be patient. Putting too much pressure on having great table manners at this age may distract the child from eating.

If your limits on what, how, or how much to eat are too rigid, there may be tremendous battles, and your child's nutrition, as well as his attitudes about food, could suffer. But the same will be true if you don't set limits. Maybe your limits at this age include 1) coming to the table with the rest of the family, 2) sitting in the chair while eating, 3) choosing what he wants from what's offered, 4) not whining or hitting, and 5) not throwing food. If such basic rules are violated, it's fine to ask your toddler to leave. (*See Chapter 5 for ideas on how to handle the diabetes side of this.*) Some parents tell their youngsters, "I warned you already that you can't scream during dinner, so you'll have to get down. But you may drink your milk before you leave if you like." Being offered this sort of choice (instead of "Drink that milk before you leave the table because I'm worried sick about you having low blood sugar!") sometimes works fairly well in getting a bit of protective carbohydrate into the child before he leaves the table.

Appetites and Schedules Change in Toddlers

Appetite is likely to be reduced during the toddler stage because growth is slowing down. Your toddler is probably growing taller, but not putting on much weight. Part of his energy needs are being met from burning his baby fat. Portion sizes for toddlers (*see Chapter 3*) are small. For example, just 16 ounces of milk and an ounce of meat give a toddler all the protein he needs in a day. With these tiny needs in mind, give a little less than you think he will eat. If he asks for more, it's his idea, and he's more likely to eat it than if you put it on the plate and then try to urge him to clean it up!

Babies are fed pretty much on their own schedule. In the toddler stage, on the other hand, your child will be joining the rest of the family in a regular schedule of meals, although snacks may be eaten on his own or with siblings or playmates. Having adequate time between meals and snacks is one important way you can help make sure that your child is actually hungry when he sits down to eat. Uncontrolled snacking between meals can reduce appetite at mealtime, and the child may refuse to eat, which can cause battles and may compromise his overall nutrition, since snacks may not include all the food groups that regular meals do.

Don't Push Sweets, Milk, or Juice

With all children, avoid making sweets and other foods into rewards.
This is just as important for the child with diabetes. Food is given even
greater emotional power when it is used as a reward. Whether you're
rewarding a child for some accomplishment or for good behavior, try
to use nonfood items like stickers, small toys, hand stamps, hugs,
kisses, or praise. These treats don't affect blood sugars and also don't
reinforce the connection between food and being rewarded. This will
pay off throughout his life in the areas of diabetes control, overall
nutrition and health, and weight maintenance.

Don't push juice and milk on your toddler. These foods are important, but in large amounts, they can compromise your child's appetite
for the other foods he needs. Toddlers should be given water to quench
thirst. Artificially sweetened drinks are safe, but some people feel that
giving them instead of water just reinforces a sweet tooth.

Insulin and Blood Glucose Monitoring in Toddlers

Insulin management in toddlers is very similar to insulin management
in infants. Short- or rapid-acting insulin is rarely used. Strong insulin
peaks are avoided as much as possible. If your child is eating in ways
that create significant blood glucose peaks, try moving the carbohydrate foods around (offer fewer choices or smaller portions when
you're trying to minimize carbohydrate) to bring down the peaks.
Many doctors prefer to delay adding meal-related insulin to the regimen until a child starts school. You can help keep postmeal blood
sugars in reasonable control by spreading carbohydrate throughout
the day. This business of trying to play food bingo to reduce the need
for meal boluses (as well as the risk for lows) is less than perfect, to
be sure.

That's why insulin pump use is growing rapidly in toddlers, as well
as in babies. The ability of pumps to give tiny, accurate amounts of
insulin for basal and bolus doses can dramatically reduce the risk for
lows. Also, insulin can be given whenever it's needed without another
needle stick.

If you're struggling to manage insulin in your very young child
with diabetes, you may want to talk to your team about the possibility
of using a pump and the specific operations of the various types avail-

able. There are now a lot of teams around the country with experience using pumps in even the youngest kids with diabetes, so this option is becoming more commonly available.

Tricks for Managing the Sticky Parts

To make shots more peaceful, give the toddler some tasks and choices to help with the process. A toddler can choose where to get the shot or wipe off the spot with a swab. Insulin can be given after the meal if your toddler's appetite or intake is unpredictable. This is not a perfect solution, especially with regular insulin. Still, even with regular, it will probably work at least as well as guessing at the dose before a child with unpredictable intake eats. It reduces parents' worries and cuts way down on mealtime battles.

Blood glucose monitoring is very important. Toddlers are still generally unable to recognize and warn you about developing lows. Test results are also vital to keeping your toddler's insulin properly adjusted to his food intake. Some of the stress around testing can now be defused because the child is getting old enough to participate more actively in the process, if he chooses. Toddlers can choose a spot to stick, pick out a lancet, or pick out a test strip from the vial.

Low blood sugars often become more of a challenge in toddlers because of their increased activity. They're so excited by this new skill of getting around on two feet that they seem to run everywhere. Providing regular meals and snacks, keeping juice readily available for treatment, and having an eye like a hawk are all helpful in cutting your toddler's risk for low blood sugar. But also make sure that your child's insulin is being managed in a way that reduces the risk for lows as much as possible: Talk with your team about pumps, insulin glargine, half-unit pens, and diluting insulin if you continue to struggle with lows and extremely variable blood sugars.

1. In infants and toddlers, the primary goal of diabetes treatment is to avoid extremely high and low blood sugar rather than to achieve near-normal blood sugars.

2. Hypoglycemia is the biggest fear of parents. Recognizing and preventing it are the biggest management challenges in very young children.

3. Symptoms of hypoglycemia can include crying, pallor, sweating, being cranky, and trembling. Symptoms are your sign to test blood sugar.

4. A small amount of a sweet liquid, such as apple juice or sugar-sweetened Kool-Aid, given by bottle or cup, is the best treatment option for little ones.

5. Either breast-feeding or bottle-feeding can provide adequate nutrition for an infant, and both are workable with diabetes control.

6. Solids are started at about four to six months of age, when babies are developmentally ready. High-carbohydrate foods (cereal, fruit, and fruit juice, for example) can be moved around in the day to help smooth out the biggest swings in blood glucose.

7. Toddlers are self-feeders and are trying hard to prove they're separate people. To minimize hassles, let them choose from the appropriate options you provide. Also offer foods in a form that helps them feed themselves.

8. Toddlers begin to move into the same meal schedule as the rest of the family.

9. Growth slows in toddlers, so energy needs and appetite may drop quite a lot. Portion sizes are likely to be quite small.

10. Don't push sweets, milk, or juice. Also, kids don't need large amounts. Too much can destroy their appetite for other foods.

11. The best tools of insulin management for infants and toddlers now include insulin pumps, half-unit pens, and diluted insulin. They can help reduce lows by better matching the tiny insulin needs of the infant and toddler.

Now she eats away from home at least as much as she eats with us.

11

Preschoolers and School-Age Children

Eleven-year-old Kate's auburn hair was the first thing most people noticed about her. It was so thick it needed special barrettes to catch it up in her preferred ponytail. And that red ponytail was bouncing as she marched into the dietitian's office. "Guess what," she said; "I must have had six carbs at lunch today. I bet my blood sugar's 300!" It wasn't the first time that Kate had been the victim of a school lunch program that didn't always deliver what the menu promised. "I know I shouldn't have eaten it all, but I was real hungry, and they didn't have any more meat or salad."

This problem came up occasionally, even though Kate and her mother dutifully reviewed the school's menus at the beginning of every month. They marked the calendar to show which days would be school lunch days and which would require a lunch from home. Some of the decisions were based on what Kate liked (chicken fingers) and disliked (beans and wieners). Others were based on

> It wasn't the first time that Kate had been the victim of a school lunch program that didn't always deliver what the menu promised.

their experience with particular meals, like the cafeteria's spaghetti, which always sent Kate's blood sugar straight to the moon.

The biggest problems happened when the cafeteria ran out of the main dish and substituted something entirely different. The substitutions weren't always great for Kate's control because she had a set dose of morning NPH covering her lunch. There was a particular amount of carbohydrate that she needed to eat each day to match that dose. Once, the cafeteria workers had offered beans and wieners in place of the promised hamburger. It might have worked, except Kate hates beans and wieners, and she didn't eat enough to cover her insulin. Predictably, she had low blood sugar that afternoon.

On the day of her visit to the dietitian, the fairly low-carbohydrate chicken finger meal had been replaced by spaghetti with marinara sauce and a roll. Kate was quite right. She had at least six carbohydrate servings, and her blood sugar was over 300 mg/dl when we tested it in the office. Her mother had spoken to the cafeteria staff about these last-minute substitutions several times, but the problem still seemed to surface occasionally. Sometimes the staff just forgot to set a meal aside for Kate before they ran out. Other times, substitute workers weren't aware of her needs. Short of sending all of Kate's meals from home, the family hadn't found a foolproof solution.

As children grow into the preschool and school-age years, they often take their first real steps out of the ever-watchful gaze of Mom and Dad. More and more of the kids' meals and activities take place away from home, where the portions or types of food can't be controlled. And the parents are also not there during gym class to notice their daughter getting pale as she runs the full length of the soccer field for the tenth time. Field trips, overnight stays at friends' homes, all-day jaunts to the mall or an amusement park; your growing child is facing choices and temptations that weren't part of the picture before. It's life. It's the way things are supposed to be. But the complications for diabetes management multiply with each new experience.

Parents are constantly trying to balance the child's need to grow and become independent against her equally important need to be safe. The process may have started even earlier, in day care. But certainly by the age of about four or five, most children are spending some time (and eating at least some meals) away from home. The frequency and the variety of these new experiences grow all through the elementary school years.

Many challenges are likely to surface for the first time between the ages of about 4 and 12. Television's influence on kids' food preferences and activity level increases tremendously. The family must deal with the need to share diabetes information with a wider circle of people. The child must be kept safe at school and in other settings, without being overprotected or singled out for unwanted attention. Reliable and acceptable ways to manage insulin and blood testing away from home must be found. Parties and sleepovers need to be managed so that diabetes doesn't interfere unduly with the child's enjoyment of normal activities. And while dealing with all these changes and challenges, it's important to promote the child's progress toward greater independence in self-care. Uncertainty is the name of the game. Every change may mean a new schedule to adjust to, a new skill to acquire, a greater need to rely on people outside the family, or a shift in responsibility between parent and child.

When you have an infant with diabetes, all her care is probably in your hands. Toddlers can begin to participate in their care in small ways—making food choices from what's offered, picking the lancet for a blood test, or choosing where to give an insulin shot, for example. Then come the preschool and school-age years, where the child develops the mental capacity and maturity to begin learning to control her own blood sugar. Your task is to help her make the transition successfully. You do this over time by sharing responsibility in ways appropriate to her development, style, and circumstances. This allows her to keep growing in independence and skill. And—of equal importance— it ensures that you stay involved so that her safety is protected until she eventually develops the maturity to take over the primary responsibility of caring for herself.

Informing Others about Your Child's Diabetes

As preschool and school-age children range farther away from home, information about her diabetes must be shared with more people. Your child's personality and acceptance of diabetes as well as the family's general communication style are factors in how comfortable she will be with this. How well she knows the people being told and how much time she spends with them are also important. Each family must decide how much, when, and who will be told. There will be some people who must know, in order to ensure your child's safety: the teacher, coach, bus driver, and the adults in any house where she will be spending a significant amount of time, for example. There may be others whom you or your child just wants to inform. The questioning and problem-solving techniques in Chapter 5 can help your family identify what's best.

Preschoolers

The preschooler is a breath of badly needed fresh air to parents who have survived the antics of the testy toddler. The two-year-old struggled against everything to prove her separateness. The three- and four-year-old defines that separateness as a happy little moon orbiting around Mom and Dad, who have become the center of the universe once again. Preschoolers are generally positive, energetic, and eager to please. They are figuring out what it means to be human, and their main way of doing that is to imitate Mom, Dad, and older siblings, so parents' food choices can strongly influence the child's choices at this age.

The preschooler's eagerness to please can help your efforts to shape her food preferences, so take advantage of it. Get the right foods into the house and onto the table. Set the meal times and rules for behavior. For the most part, the preschooler will go along with the program. If she strays, refuses, or makes mistakes, just say no. Be polite but firm. Don't make it personal, and avoid shame and guilt. Because your approval and good opinion are so important to her, she's likely to go along with you most of the time, provided these things do not become a battleground. Notice it and congratulate her when she tries to do the right thing. If you criticize her efforts, she may stop trying altogether because she doesn't want to disappoint or anger you. If she's afraid to make mistakes (in food choices or table manners, for example), she'll have trouble learning what she needs to. Mistakes are part of the learning process.

A preschooler's limited attention span and need to explore go hand in hand with her inability to sit still for very long. Expect a preschooler to eat with gusto and focus for just about as long as she's actually hungry. After that, she's likely to dawdle or want to head off on other pursuits.

Her imagination is developing rapidly, and she may have difficulty distinguishing between real and make-believe. Logical, critical thinking comes later, so she can't always make the connection between her actions and their consequences, which is one of the reasons why Mom and Dad still need to be in charge of meals and snacks. At this age, a child simply doesn't think ahead to the probable consequences of skipping a snack or playing harder than usual.

Eating Style

The shape, texture, size, and color of the food offered to the preschooler are very important. She will accept moist foods more readily than things that are dry or tough because they're easier to chew and swallow. Cut her food into manageable pieces, but be aware of shapes, because she may be. Anyone who has ever cut a peanut butter sandwich into little squares for a three-year-old who was expecting triangles has learned this important lesson! Because of their stage of mental development, most preschoolers don't really grasp that a given food cut up into different shapes is still the same food. They focus on what they see, and squares are different from triangles. Logic will get you nowhere.

Table manners and food-handling skills improve slowly but surely through the preschool years, but they still don't reach real mastery. A five-year-old can probably get through dinner without spilling the milk. But he may still have trouble managing a knife and fork. When setting expectations for mealtime behavior, take your child's level of coordination into account. Expecting more than the child is capable of will increase everybody's stress level. And it still won't make a five-year-old as coordinated as an eight-year-old.

Structured Meals and Snacks

Having diabetes in the family tends to keep everyone tuned in to the importance of regularly scheduled meals and snacks, and this meets the preschooler's needs beautifully. If you plan and schedule defined meals and snacks, you help your child develop a more predictable pattern of hunger and satisfaction, and she will eat more consistently and willingly. This can be a big aid to diabetes control. To help ensure that she has an appetite for meals when they're offered, limit snacks to the scheduled ones as much as possible. Make sure that there's enough time between meals and snacks to allow her to get hungry. Avoid juice, milk, or other caloric beverages between meals and snacks, and offer water instead.

What if your child begs for more food right after a meal? If she ate her meal and is still hungry, giving her more food is probably the right thing to do. To promote blood sugar control without creating the need for another shot, you could offer things that are less likely to raise blood sugar: nuts, peanut butter on celery, beef jerky sticks, low-fat cheese, or other low-carbohydrate items. But if the child refused the previous meal (even though some choices were available and the consequences of not eating were explained), it's may be best to take a harder line. Kids need to learn to live with the fallout of their actions, whether it is being hungry until snack time or having low blood sugar. Letting this kind of situation play out at home is a safe and responsible way to help your child learn the importance of eating regular meals and snacks. (As we've explained before, this is especially important if she uses regular or NPH to cover meals. Snacks are needed to prevent lows because of the broad peaks of these insulins.)

Letting a child experience first hand what happens when she refuses to eat is more effective and less stressful than trying to force her to eat. When the consequence comes, the teachable moment is at hand. It is an effective approach that can be used even with preschoolers in many areas of behavior.

A child who picked at her meal and later comes panhandling for an extra snack could also be offered her leftovers from the previous meal. This prevents kids thinking they can fish around for something better if they refuse a meal.

Insulin and Blood Sugar Monitoring in Preschoolers

Insulin and testing regimens for preschoolers tend to remain much like the toddler's. Sensitivity to rapid-acting and regular insulin remains high, largely because of the child's small body size. Proportions for meal boluses are likely to be less than the approximately 50 percent of total insulin that older kids and adults would get. Blood sugar monitoring continues to be important, not only for glucose control, but also for peace of mind. Eating may be low or erratic at times, and the child may still be unable to always recognize low blood sugar and tell you about it. (*See also insulin, blood testing, and insulin pumps in Chapter 10.*)

School-Age Children

There's a reason why formal schooling starts at around age six or seven. This marks the child's passage into the realm of rational, concrete thought. Tremendous learning took place earlier, to be sure: walking, speaking, social skills, coordination, and so on. With that background and a reasonable command of the language, the school-age child is ready to learn about the wider world. Her curiosity is tremendous. Her social interests become directed outside the family. She is able to follow rational lines of thought and appreciate cause and effect. As a result, she can begin to accept responsibility for her own actions.

Most youngsters become physically able to perform the majority of diabetes self-care tasks by about age 10, but emotions and maturity are still not at an adult level. Parents must stay involved in daily care and make sure diabetes management doesn't suffer. During the school years, her ability to recognize and inform you about developing hypoglycemia should become well tuned. She probably can select and administer her own treatment for mild low blood sugar episodes. She can understand the effects of various foods on her blood sugar and make appropriate food choices, even when Mom hasn't laid out all the right foods in all the right portions. She won't make the best choices all the time. The lure of being just like her friends, eating foods she may never get at home, or just not thinking about it for once is sometimes too powerful. But she can understand the likely outcome of her choices, and she can learn from the experience.

Catching her doing something right and praising her for it encourages good behavior. It's important to acknowledge her effort, even when the outcome isn't everything you might want. Doing the blood test is important, regardless of whether you like the result. Riding her bike after school instead of zoning out in front of the computer is great, even if it causes low blood sugar.

Try out new ways to deal with the challenges of the school-age years. Whether these experiments turn out well or not, they're the best way to learn. Keep talking with your school-age child about her diabetes management. Ask her what's working and what's not, what she wants, and what bothers her about her diabetes. Stay involved in the process and try to convey a positive, supportive outlook. This helps your child do the same.

It will also pay big dividends when your child becomes a teenager. Anything that has been an earlier source of stress or hard feelings is likely to explode into a full-blown battle during the teen years. If you have been able to establish a comfortable, cooperative approach to diabetes management while the child is younger, the upheaval may be less when puberty strikes.

School Lunch

Children with diabetes eat school lunches, just like other kids. Sometimes they like it, and sometimes they don't, just like other kids. Parents have found a variety of ways to manage the problems unique to diabetes management, with varying levels of cooperation or action from the school. The basic approach is to review the menus with your child, selecting the meals that the child likes and that are in tune with your nutrition preferences. Most parents seem to use a combination of fine-tuning the insulin doses to handle anticipated portion sizes and having the child try to control how much is actually eaten. This is obviously more realistic with older school-age kids than with very young ones. Any needed modifications are worked out while the parent and child review the menus.

One mom we work with had isolated three school lunch meals that always seemed to send her son's blood sugar too high: spaghetti, pizza, and chicken stir-fry. She discussed it with her son, and they were able to agree on some changes he could make on-site. They agreed that he would not eat the garlic bread with the spaghetti, eat only two of the three pizza slices, and leave at least half a cup of the rice uneaten on the plate when he had the stir-fry. The youngster preferred doing this, since he hated being singled out to get different foods than his friends and bringing lunch from home. Obviously, his lunch was being covered by a set dose of intermediate-acting insulin (NPH in his case), and the food needed to be kept in sync with the dose. Even for kids who are perfectly capable of adjusting rapid-acting insulin for food, this option seems to be pretty rarely used for school days. School policies that forbid having medicines, let alone needles, in a child's possession at school are widespread.

Some parents tell us they've been able to convince lunchroom personnel to standardize their child's servings to exchange-size (or calorie point or whatever system) portions. This is a matter of the parents' style, how the child feels about the extra attention, and the willingness of the school staff to do it. However, we think that it eventually serves the child better for her to learn how to manage this kind of situation herself. After all, it's what happens in restaurants and at friends' homes. Learning how to handle it—whether by deciding how much to eat of what's offered or by adjusting the insulin dose to cover the meal—is a key skill.

Reviewing menus and trying to monitor portion sizes for consistency are helpful. But they do not necessarily ensure that lunch at school will go smoothly. One possible problem that can come up—unscheduled food substitutions—is described at the beginning of the chapter. Another cause of difficulties is odd lunch schedules. This doesn't seem to be an issue everywhere, but in some localities it's quite a hassle. Usually beginning in middle school or high school, kids' lunch periods may be scheduled as early as 10:30 A.M. or as late as 1:30 P.M.

For a child on morning NPH or Lente, these kinds of odd schedules can create quite a challenge. For example, one 12-year-old seventh grader who took his morning rapid-acting insulin and NPH with breakfast at about 7:45 A.M. was assigned to the 10:45 A.M. lunch period. That was just too early to be eating a big lunch on his insulin regimen. Working with their team, he and his parents decided to switch to regular insulin for breakfast coverage on school days and reduce his morning NPH so he didn't go low in the afternoon. Lunch turned out to be nothing much more than a heavy snack, since Todd really wasn't hungry enough to eat a full lunch at 10:45 A.M. anyway. He ate a sandwich at his desk at around 1:00 P.M. and another snack after school. Other families might have chosen to work with the school to get the schedule changed. But factors other than diabetes are often involved in these decisions, like class schedules, the school's flexibility, or the child's desires to stay with friends. It's trying to balance all the priorities that can get to be such a challenge!

When lunch periods are scheduled too late in relation to a set morning insulin dose, there are a couple of options that might help. A snack containing carbohydrate, protein, and fat (a half or whole sandwich, for example) can be eaten at the old lunchtime to tide the child over until the late lunch period. Or the morning NPH or Lente insulin dose can be reduced, and an injection of rapid-acting insulin can be added at the time of the late lunch, but the child must be willing and able to take the extra injection at school. This can be made much simpler by using an insulin pen rather than a syringe and vial. School policy plays a big role in how well this would work for you.

Diabetes Care at School

Children with diabetes in the United States have the right to care for their diabetes at school. The Individuals with Disability Education Act (IDEA) and Section 504 of the Rehabilitation Act of 1973 guarantee this right. These laws prohibit discrimination against children with "disabilities," including diabetes. Parents can use these laws, if necessary, to ensure that their children with diabetes can care for their medical needs while taking part in school activities. Any school that receives federal funding is subject to the IDEA and Section 504 laws. (A School Bill of Rights for Children with Diabetes is shown in Table 11.1.)

If your child's school isn't providing these things, you should first educate the school administration, teacher, and other key personnel. Make sure they understand the laws and your child's needs. Schools that still refuse to cooperate should be advised that you are requesting preparation of an Individualized Education Program (IEP) and a Section 504 accommodation for your child. Not all parents want to file a so-called 504 plan. They resent their child being identified as disabled. But it is an option you should be aware of. Once you request a plan, the school must meet with you to negotiate how they will meet your

TABLE 11.1 School Bill of Rights for Children with Diabetes

Children with diabetes require medical care to remain healthy. The need for medical care does not end while the child is at school. Thus, while at school, each child with diabetes must be allowed to:

1. Do blood sugar checks
2. Treat hypoglycemia with emergency sugar
3. Inject insulin when necessary
4. Eat snacks when necessary
5. Eat lunch at an appropriate time and have enough time to finish the meal
6. Have free and unrestricted access to water and the bathroom
7. Participate fully in physical education (gym class) and extracurricular activities, including field trips

Source: Childrenwithdiabetes.com

child's needs. If you still can't negotiate a suitable plan, you can file a complaint with your state's department of education. More information about the legal aspects of diabetes care in the school can be found on the Children with Diabetes web site (*www.childrenwithdiabetes. com*). It would be great if such extreme measures were never necessary.

Management Options at School

Making sure that your child's diabetes is managed appropriately at school is important to your peace of mind and to her well-being. Your child's teachers, principal, school nurse (if you're lucky enough to still have one!), school secretary, food service personnel, and bus driver all need some level of diabetes knowledge to ensure her safety. Some of the topics that are helpful to touch on are listed in Table 11.2. You or your child may want to do the honors, or you might do it together. Guidelines and literature to help you with this important task are available

TABLE 11.2 Information Needed by School Personnel

- What diabetes is and isn't (contagious!)
- Care that may/must be done at school
- Low blood glucose (only emergency likely to happen at school)
  Causes
  Symptoms
  Treatment
  What to do if the child refuses to eat
- High blood sugar
  Child's need to drink and go to bathroom
  When to call the parents
- Meals/school lunch
- Snacks
  What
  When
  How you'll provide them
- Gym class
- Parties
- On the bus
- After-school punishment
- Informing substitute teachers

from the American Diabetes Association and at www.childrenwith diabetes.com. In addition, some local chapters of the American Association of Diabetes Educators can provide training programs conducted by certified diabetes educators for school personnel. A meeting with all the relevant school staff at the beginning of the year makes sense if you can get the cooperation of the school and the individuals involved.

Don't try to make school personnel into "diabetes police," expecting them to control what your child eats or report to you the specific details of each day. They probably don't have the time, and your child won't appreciate being singled out in that way. Obviously, school personnel should be asked to inform you of anything unusual that happens, but being a member of the diabetes police is not part of the cafeteria lady's job description.

Virtually every family struggles with how much testing will be done at school. Before lunch and before gym class are desirable times, but not everyone can manage to get them done. Testing when low blood sugar is suspected is always a priority. This can be more of a challenge for a child who's too young to do a test independently. Who will help her, and when and where will they do it?

It's important to ask how your child feels about testing at school before deciding what to ask for. Sometimes, testing is not much of a hassle: Testing materials are kept in the classroom, and the child and the teacher work out an acceptable and nondisruptive routine. Other times, school policies or the individual teachers or staff members involved make it a tremendous hassle. At some schools, for example, testing materials must be kept in the counselor's or nurse's office, which requires pulling the child out of class and making the test more visible and disruptive (not to mention risky, if the child is low). If your child must go to a different location to test at school, make sure a companion goes with her when she's feeling low. If you elect to file a 504 plan, include this important safety precaution (although some schools do this automatically).

Parties

There are many ways to successfully manage parties, whether away or at home. There's the "control the environment" school of thought in which parents try to see to it that "offending" foods, such as sweets, are simply not available. This is not an easy or a popular approach, and we think it delays the child's learning how to manage sweets right along with other carbohydrate foods. Still, some families use it, and not only for diabetes-related reasons. Some folks restrict sweets on general nutritional grounds. Another strategy is to feed oatmeal or lentils (high in soluble fiber) at breakfast to help blunt the effect of eating sweets at school parties. This probably works best if the party happens during the morning hours. Another possibility is adjusting the insulin upward, after negotiating beforehand the type and amount of extra food she will be eating at the party. Some families simply encourage the child to enjoy the party and then touch up the blood sugars as necessary afterward. None of these options will produce perfect blood sugar control, but that's OK. The child with diabetes needs to have fun, celebrate, and be a part of the group. That's as important to overall growth and development as blood sugar control is to physical health.

Overnight Stays with Friends

Having sleepovers at your house is sometimes the perfect answer, especially at younger ages. Besides making you very popular with the other parents, this is about the easiest way to give you and your child what each one wants. You get things important to your peace of mind: 1) no food surprises, 2) observation of what's going on, 3) appreciation of what happens to appetite and blood sugar when eight-year-olds stay awake giggling all night, and 4) assurance that neither the bedtime nor morning insulin will be forgotten in the shuffle. And your child gets to enjoy her friends' company with your full support.

After doing this a few times, you will have a good idea of what it takes to handle a sleepover, which will make it much easier to prepare for that first sleepover at someone else's house, when the time comes. Obviously, the cooperation of the hosting parent is important. Ideally, it will be a parent who already has some experience dealing with your child's diabetes on shorter visits. But this may not be possible. Many parents today use cell phones and beepers to ensure everyone's comfort and safety. With Mom and Dad only a speed-dial button away, help and advice will be there when questions or problems arise.

Fast Food

Fast food is a familiar feature of the eating landscape for most families and children. Fast food is convenient, relatively inexpensive, tasty, and—probably most important—expertly advertised. Many people deplore this trend, whether it's because of the depletion of the rain forest to make grazing room for all those ill-fated cattle or of fast foods' generally high content of fat and sodium. In spite of these and other concerns, Americans eat at franchise food chains an average of seven times a week. So we accept the inevitability of fast foods—the trick is to know and compensate for their shortcomings while capitalizing their one advantage for diabetes management: consistent, known portion sizes.

Many fast foods are high in fat and salt, although lower fat choices are available at most of the larger chains. Choose grilled meat sandwiches instead of fried. Stick with the plainer burgers instead of the double-meat, double-cheese varieties. At McDonald's, you can get a salad and low-fat dressing, and at Wendy's a bowl of chili. But these may not be a hit with younger kids.

Fat can really add up when a whole meal is chosen off the fast-food menu, especially if you choose a larger sandwich and "super-size" the fries, but fat and salt can be minimized through either item choice or portion size. For example, a burger, fries, and diet soda is a pretty standard fast-food meal or snack. Combining the burger with a side salad with low-fat dressing instead of fries will greatly reduce the fat and salt content of the meal. However, it's probably more realistic for kids to simply choose the regular size fries instead of the super size. And it will make quite a difference. The super size of fries at some chains is a full *three times* the size of the regular fries. That usually means six carbs and a boatload of fat. If your child wants or needs more carbohydrate than the regular fries provide, consider bringing fruit from home to round out the meal. This can get the job done and provide a few stray vitamins and minerals (and less fat) in the process. This is a great idea from a nutritional viewpoint because most fast food meals lack fruits and vegetables anyway.

If your child eats fast food frequently, it's a good idea to make these adjustments routinely. But if fast foods are just an occasional treat, it's probably fine to let her eat her favorites along with her friends. Limiting fat and salt is not really necessary in the short term for most kids, unless they already have blood pressure or blood fat problems. But this is when lifelong food habits and preferences are set. It's probably best to encourage less fat, less salt, and more fruits and vegetables most of the time so that the kids grow up eating that way. The exchange values and carbohydrate, fat, and sodium content of most fast foods are readily available in literature produced by all the major chains.

For all their shortcomings, fast foods have one enormous advantage when it comes to diabetes control: their consistency. Franchise food operations are generally obsessive about portion sizes. Say you sell a couple of million bean burritos a year. If everybody gets an extra ounce of beans on their burrito, it cuts way into your profit margin. That's the main reason employees are trained to make each item consistently. Once you and your child figure out how to fit a given fast-food item into the management plan—either by substituting for other foods in a set meal plan or by adjusting insulin doses—you're set. Fast food is simply not a wild card anymore, like the lasagna or cookies at a friend's house, where ingredients and portion sizes are often unknowable.

Kid-Style Diabetes Education

If your child was diagnosed at a younger age, any diabetes education that took place was probably directed at you. Now that she's reached school age, however, she's old enough to benefit from diabetes education on her own. It should be suited to her age and interest. At this age, children are eager to learn about their world and master the skills required for living in it successfully. Knowing more about their diabetes can give them a greater sense of mastery, reducing stress and improving confidence. Diabetes camp is a great place for this type of learning. You might also ask around in your community for classes geared specifically to kids. There should be games, activities, a lot of discussion about what it feels like to have diabetes, and a minimum of lecture about facts and figures. The KidZone section of the American Diabetes Association webpage (http://www.diabetes.org) has kid-friendly information. There are also quite a few good books about diabetes written for kids of various ages. Ask your team which ones they recommend (besides *Sweet Kids*, of course!).

THE BOTTOM LINE

1. Preschool and school-age children cannot be under constant parental supervision, so a major focus during these years must be to help children learn to control their own blood sugars. This includes learning to choose from a wider variety of foods and doing enough blood testing to see the effect.

2. There is an increased need to inform other people about the child's diabetes.

3. Preschoolers are eager to please, which can help you shape good eating habits.

4. Regular meals and snacks help control appetite and improve nutritional intake. They can also play an important role in diabetes control, especially when set insulin doses are used.

5. Review school lunch menus with your child when they are published. Decide when she will get school lunch and, if necessary, how she will modify it.

6. Work with school personnel to ensure that diabetes care gets the appropriate type and amount of attention. Educate and negotiate. Consider filing a 504 plan if you have difficulties getting what your child needs.

7. Diabetes needn't stop your child from enjoying the same activities as her friends. Parties, overnight stays with buddies, and eating out at fast-food places can all be managed without sacrificing diabetes control.

12

I keep taking more and more insulin, but my blood sugars aren't getting any better. Mom and Dad think I'm cheating like crazy, and we fight about it a lot.

Teenagers

Adam had been a fixture at diabetes camp every summer since his diabetes was diagnosed at the age of eight. He was a very bright kid, at home with all the diabetes routines. And he had a sweet, quiet way that won him many friends. At 13, he seemed like a natural choice to become a junior counselor.

But when he arrived for the first day of camp, we wondered if we'd made a mistake. In the year since we'd last seen him, Adam's light brown sporty haircut had been replaced by a spiky crop of jet-black hair. His jacket, clunky boots, and sweatshirt all matched his inky hair; baggy shorts, a silver nose ring, and a couple of tattoos completed the startling makeover. He definitely had blossomed into full adolescence. Some of the staff wondered out loud if he would be a good influence on the younger campers. We shouldn't have worried.

Under the unique garb was the same sweet Adam. The littlest kids barely seemed to notice his appearance, and a pack of them were con-

Adam's diabetes control had exploded right along with his surging adolescent hormones.

stantly trailing him. The older ones pronounced his nose ring either "cool!" or "gross!" and then everyone got on with the business of having a good time. But besides his appearance, something else about Adam had changed since the previous year. His diabetes control had exploded right along with his surging adolescent hormones. This smart kid who seemed to have such a lock on his diabetes in the past was now struggling, with little success, to control his soaring blood sugars. He admitted that he was relieved to be at camp, where he could escape the arguments that had been raging between him and his parents nearly every day.

"I know I'm not always as careful as I used to be, but I swear I'm not being this bad," he complained as he tossed his record book to the nurse. "My parents are sure it's something I'm doing that's got things so messed up. I wonder if it would actually be any worse if I just blew it all off . . . the food, the testing, the whole thing. I don't even want to write down my numbers anymore, because I know what's going to happen when Mom and Dad see them."

Growth, Hormones, and Diabetes Control

Adolescence is a time of huge changes, both emotional and physical. Living through those changes is enough of a challenge for most mere mortals. But things can be even worse when the teen has diabetes. Phenomenal growth and raging hormones often have a huge impact on diabetes control. Adam and his frustrated parents were right in the middle of it. Rising levels of several hormones—especially growth hormones—work against insulin, making it less effective. Glucose control gets harder to achieve and the need for insulin increases.

We used to think control worsened during the teen years solely because of looser self-care. We now know that's only part of the story. A major factor is that nature itself is working against control in growing teens. Keep this in mind the next time you're tempted to lose your temper over your teenager's blood sugar results. Insulin requirements will probably remain well above normal while your teen is growing—twice the previous dose is not unusual. Insulin doses and blood sugar levels usually fall back to more expected levels once growth is complete.

Emotional Change and Development

All this is happening at the worst possible time. The typical behavior of adolescents—testing boundaries, taking risks, seeking identity—means that structured treatment plans are often ignored. Many parents react to the loss of blood sugar control and to the teen's provocative behavior by becoming more controlling. Unfortunately, this generally makes the teen dig in his heels more firmly. Family relationships take a beating and, when they do, everybody loses.

Every teen must learn who he is and gain independence. In fact, these are the main tasks of this stage of his life. As important and predictable as it is, however, a teenager's efforts to master these tasks can put diabetes care at risk. This is especially likely if parents respond by going to extremes: trying to control the diabetes themselves or giving up completely and handing it all over to the teenager. The first extreme is impossible to maintain: No young adult will tolerate his parents' efforts to manage his diabetes forever. Either openly or in secret, he will take control in the only way possible under the circumstances—by refusing to cooperate. The second extreme is also full of risk: Important self-care tasks will probably be neglected because few teens are prepared to fly solo when it comes to diabetes care.

The trick is to stay involved without being overbearing. If responsibility is gradually shifted from parent to teen, with parents continuing to participate in some supportive, mutually agreed upon way, blood sugar control can be maintained. Try to look on the inevitable mistakes as learning opportunities. Ask lots of questions that help your teen think through what happened. ("Wow. That's a high one, Chad. What do you think might have caused it?") Get him to talk about how he was affected by the outcome. ("How were you feeling then?" or, "Tell me about what happened.") Ask him how he might use what he learned to produce a better outcome in the future.

And don't criticize what he eats! Doing so only hands him a script for getting your goat. Remember that teens need to test boundaries. Teenagers whose food choices are criticized tend to skip more meals and have worse overall nutrition than those whose families take a more relaxed approach do. Those pesky job descriptions again: You get the right stuff on the table and leave the choices in the kids' hands. Of course, teens have access to many foods that you haven't chosen. But the basic premise remains true.

A relaxed, philosophical approach is especially important for parents during the teen years. We need to 1) accept that blood sugar goals should probably be relaxed to some extent, especially during growth spurts and when your teen is uncooperative, and 2) remember that

adolescence will end some day. If you and your child are still friendly at
the end of it and you have managed to avoid major problems with his
diabetes, you all deserve a huge pat on the back.

The Time for Independent Doctor Visits

Adolescence is a good time for your kid to start seeing the doctor and
educator on her own, but that doesn't mean that you should become
totally uninvolved. It's another case of finding a middle road that
meets both your needs. You will still occasionally want to join her
during visits, or you may want to go together, with some time set aside
for her to see the healthcare provider alone. Most teens welcome the
privacy, and it's important because it encourages frank talk about
subjects that need to be discussed, such as sex and drinking.

Separate medical visits signal your trust in her developing ability
to take care of herself. And they are an important step in learning to
relate to and communicate with a health professional on her own.
When she starts college, goes to work, or moves to another city, she will
need that skill. If she begins the process while she's still at home, you
can talk about how it's going and can help if needed. You might want
to ask the team for summary reports of the visits—excluding any con-
fidential information—so you can stay in the loop while still respecting
her privacy and independence.

The Importance of Peer Relationships

Peer relationships become the major focus of most kids' lives at this
age. Family ties may take a backseat to friendships. At times, teens seem
to have only two goals: to be as different from their parents as possible
and to be as much like their friends as possible. Because his friends are
so important, your child probably wants to do whatever they do. This
helps him feel comfortable and secure. If his friends dress all in black
and listen to stuff you don't consider to be music, it may irritate you,
but it doesn't really affect diabetes care (or anything else important, for
that matter). On the other hand, if the friends hang around the mall
eating pizza after school, your teen will probably want to do the same.
In this case, the impact on diabetes control could be substantial.

Making an issue of these things, especially in ways that your teen
experiences as critical or nagging, usually escalates the battle. And you

probably won't get what you want anyway! In fact, diabetes self-care and control may get worse. When you throw down the gauntlet, you hand your teen a perfect tool for resisting your authority—an essential part of every teenager's job description. Try to keep diabetes care out of the fray as much as possible. You can best do this by not criticizing his self-care efforts, even when sorely tempted. Instead, use the questioning and problem-solving approach first described in Chapter 5.

One of us sometimes makes a deal with teens who are struggling against both their parents and their diabetes: "If you're looking for a way to get your parents' goat, look someplace other than your diabetes. Pierce your nose. Dye your hair blue. Get a tattoo. But promise me you won't skip your insulin. That's just too risky." This worked well for many years until the day an irate father called and said, "My son says he dyed his hair blue because you told him he could! How could you do such a thing?" That one took some explaining!

Crazy Schedules

Few teens these days follow regular schedules. An early morning job one day and after-school activities the next can make may make the diabetes routine a real challenge. For most young adults, the days of laying out the after-school snack and being able to count on when you'll get it are gone. Snacks, if they're eaten at all, may be coming from different sources and at different times on different days of the week.

Gina's schedule was pretty typical. Her mom's happiest day came when Gina got her driver's license. That meant Mom could stop driving the busy high school junior to her many after-school activities. On Monday, Gina grabbed a small hamburger and a diet soda at a fast-food place on her way to ballet class. Tuesday, she stayed at school for cheerleading practice, so she had to remember to bring something from home because the snack bar was closed after school. Wednesday, she needed to bring less of a snack because she was sitting down all afternoon, working on the yearbook. Thursday, she went home after school and could fix her own snack when she got there. What she ate depended on whether she was staying home to study or heading back out with friends. Friday night, she usually had a ball game to attend. She needed to make sure that her snack and dinner were pretty substantial, since the cheerleading she did at the games really lowered her blood sugar. Usually, it was another fast-food night.

Staying Up All Night and Sleeping Late

One of the schedule problems that often surfaces during adolescence involves late nights and the even later mornings that follow them. Staying up late does not necessarily affect insulin needs or diabetes control. The teen who stays up all night studying, reading, or watching TV may not see much of a difference in his blood sugar unless he's also eating extra snacks without taking extra insulin to compensate.

But when a teen is staying out late doing more active things, the effect on control can be dramatic. To complicate matters, a teenager may be out dancing (and lowering blood sugar), eating extra food (raising blood sugar), or drinking alcohol (increasing risk for low blood sugar), all in the same evening. The only reasonable way to approach these situations is with an open mind and a lot of blood glucose test strips. Testing before and after going out provides the information you and your teen will need to start identifying patterns. Of course, the more details you know (how much dancing, what kind of food, how many beers, and so on), the more meaningful the blood glucose results will be. History is a great teacher, but only if enough information was gathered to understand what happened.

Teens who want to sleep late—and are there any who don't?—can face a real challenge, depending on how their insulin therapy is being managed. If the background insulin is coming from a pump or bed-time Lantus (the once-daily peakless insulin), sleeping late in the morning is not a problem. When the basal rate on a pump or the bed-time dose of Lantus is set correctly, there is no need for a timely shot in the morning to keep the background insulin at an appropriate level. Blood sugars stay stable while the teen snoozes. When he gets up and is ready to eat, he takes a premeal dose of rapid-acting insulin to compensate.

Those who aren't on the pump or Lantus have other considerations as they plan for this situation. The morning dose of any background insulin that is taken more than once a day (NPH, Lente, or perhaps Ultralente) must be taken reasonably close to the prescribed time. If it isn't, the insulin level may drop so low that the liver starts releasing glucose, causing the first blood sugar of the day to be sky high. There may be urine ketones as well. In addition, they can't wake up in the morning, take their usual premeal insulin dose, and then go back to bed without eating, since this might lead to a low blood sugar reaction. A workable plan for those still taking two injections of background insulin a day might be to wake up, take the regular dose of background insulin, and then eat a small snack before going back to sleep. The pen or syringe and snack could be set on the bedside table next to the alarm clock the night before. Not a perfect plan, but workable.

A flexible insulin regimen that provides the right level of background insulin between meals and overnight, and boluses of rapid-acting insulin at meals, will give most teens the best results. The background insulin dose is correct when blood sugar neither rises nor falls much when food isn't eaten. If they have to eat meals at specific times to prevent lows, the background insulin dose is too high at that time. If blood sugars rise when they haven't eaten anything, the background insulin has fallen too low. Once the background insulin is right, then sleeping in, delaying, or even skipping meals becomes possible. When the routine changes, extra blood tests are still needed to make sure things are working as planned, but at least a measure of freedom and spontaneity is possible.

Teen Appetites and Calorie Needs

Many teenagers have huge appetites. Most adults would consider a hamburger, fries, and a diet soda a reasonably sized meal. The teen may want twice that amount. They also eat more snacks. Because they're burning calories rapidly, they tend to get hungry often. Any time substantial amounts of food are eaten without a corresponding peak of insulin, high blood sugar will be the result. Flexible basal/bolus insulin plans usually match teens' hectic schedules and eating habits best, and pumps, pens, and rapid-acting insulin for meal coverage are the most flexible tools for this. Teens need these options for "touching up" insulin when extra food is eaten.

Here is an example of a typical challenge encountered on less flexible insulin plans. Perhaps your teen, who is on two shots daily, wants to eat fast food after school with his friends. And you want his blood sugar to be somewhere near planet Earth before dinner. Some fast-food choices would minimize the rise in blood glucose (chicken nuggets instead of a big sandwich, or maybe taking it easy on the fries). Increasing the morning NPH insulin would also provide better coverage, but this locks him into eating a large snack. If he changed his mind about the snack, his blood sugar would be low. An additional small bolus of rapid-acting insulin, taken with the fast food, could also keep blood sugars in check. This would be more convenient and less conspicuous if he had an insulin pen, instead of a syringe and vial. (And easier still with a pump.) This is not cheating, this is "playing pancreas." If your child didn't have diabetes and was eating that food, his body would put out extra insulin to cover it.

Worries about Big Appetites. When calorie needs are high, enormous meals may not cause unwanted weight gain, especially if the teen is large, growing, physically active, and male. All of these factors greatly increase energy needs. A 17-year-old girl who has stopped growing probably would need much less food than a 17-year-old boy of similar size would. (Boys generally have larger muscle mass, and muscles use more calories per pound than other types of body tissue.)

The amount of food that it takes to meet most teens' nutrient needs (for protein, vitamins, minerals, and so on) is much less than the amount of food it takes to meet their energy needs. That's why most teens can eat potato chips, French fries, pizza, and ice cream—which provide relatively little nutrition for their high calories—without gaining weight. With their high fat content, these foods aren't exactly the stuff of a dietitian's dreams, but they are a reality of many teens' diets. And they can be consumed without causing unwanted weight gain when calorie needs are high enough.

If you're worried that your child is eating too much, there are ways to tell if your child is eating the right amount of food (*see also Chapter 2*). If weight is normal and diabetes control is reasonable, chances are that the amount of food is just what your child needs to fuel the current growth spurt. But keep in mind that a child with diabetes may lose or maintain weight, even if he's eating more than he needs, when blood sugar control is poor. Sugar and all the calories it contains leave the body in large quantities. And if a child eats more than he needs and follows it with insulin to keep blood sugar in check, he will gain weight, just like people who don't have diabetes. (*If you are concerned about eating problems and disorders, see Chapter 9.*)

Alcohol, Driving, Tobacco, Drugs, and Sex

Experimenting with alcohol, drugs, and sex is common in teens. Statistics tell us that kids who engage in one or more of these behaviors, at least occasionally, greatly outnumber those who don't. We might wish that this were not so, but it is, and we have to face it. If you can discuss these topics with your teen in a reasonably comfortable and non-accusing fashion, do it; if you can't, another responsible adult should.

Alcohol. Pure alcohol does not raise blood glucose. The body handles alcohol very much like fat, so some healthcare providers recommend that people with diabetes exchange alcohol for fat in the meal plan. We don't recommend this because if a teen is going to drink (which is not only illegal but also probably disapproved of by his parents), we don't think he's going to bother counting exchanges while he's doing it. Furthermore, it's not necessary. Pure alcohol has no effect on blood sugar, so people with type 1 diabetes can just add modest amounts of alcohol to their food intake without raising blood sugar or increasing their need for insulin. By "modest" we mean up to two drinks, if a drink is understood to be a 12-ounce beer, a glass of wine, or an ounce of distilled liquor.

More alcohol than this won't raise blood sugar directly, but it could still affect it. People who drink a lot tend to ignore their self-care. They are less aware of what they're eating, they may forget to take insulin on time, and so on. Also, because alcohol raises the risk for hypoglycemia, heavy drinking gets quite risky—even riskier for the diabetic teen than for someone else.

While the body is processing alcohol, it is unable to release sugar from the liver if it's needed. In addition, alcohol increases the efficiency of whatever insulin is already in the body. So someone with type 1 diabetes who is drinking is more likely to have not only a low blood sugar reaction but a severe one, because the body is not able to respond normally to the falling glucose level.

Unless someone actually gives a teen the facts about alcohol and diabetes, he is likely to make some dangerous assumptions. Many kids lump sweets and alcohol together, because they were told at some point to stay away from both. He may skip a meal when he's experimenting with alcohol, which may seem like a good way to compensate. Instead, he ends up putting himself at high risk for hypoglycemia.

Since drinking is a distinct possibility from at least junior high school on, kids from about the age of 12 need to have the straight scoop on alcohol. In addition to the facts about hypoglycemia risk described here and in Chapter 7, they should know at least the following guidelines:

- If you're going to drink, keep the amounts small. Up to two drinks can probably be added to your normal diet with relatively little effect on blood sugar.
- Because of the risk for low blood sugar, never skip meals when drinking alcohol.
- Choose light beers, dry wines, or distilled liquor, and use noncaloric mixers. The carbohydrate in sweeter drinks and mixers may raise blood sugar. Insulin can be adjusted to compensate for this, but it can get complicated when paired with the hypoglycemic effect of the alcohol itself.
- Wear a diabetes medical I.D. at all times, but especially when drinking. Others (friends, police) might confuse a low blood sugar reaction for drunkenness if you've been drinking, and fail to treat you or call for help.
- Make sure someone in your group knows about your diabetes and what to do about low blood sugar. This is always important, but even more so if you're drinking alcohol.

Driving. Getting a driver's license is a big day in a teen's life. But it's a double-antacid day for most parents. It's hard to feel confident about your 16-year-old piloting several tons of steel through busy streets when you've watched him walk into walls because he wasn't paying attention. When the teen in question has diabetes, the stresses are multiplied. In addition to all the usual concerns, the teen with diabetes has hypoglycemia to consider. And the risk is real. Blood sugars can drop when your child is behind the wheel, just as they can at any other time, and he could seriously harm both himself and others if low blood sugar slows his thinking or responses. And of course, drinking and driving is an especially dangerous combination for the teen with diabetes.

This is one of those areas that cry out for good communication, questioning, and problem solving. Teens want to drive. Parents want them to be safe. Mutually acceptable guidelines for eating, drinking, testing, and driving are needed if both sets of desires are going to be fulfilled.

Tobacco. Some teens try smoking or chewing tobacco because everybody else is doing it, or because it makes them feel grown up. Once started, they are hard habits to break, and their potential for harm grows the longer they're continued. They have little or no effect on blood glucose control, but they do impair circulation and greatly increase the risk for heart disease and cancer.

These health risks rarely stop tobacco use, however. Teens who smoke or chew need to know about these risks, but it's hard to sell kids on a long-term issue like cancer risk or an "old people's" problem like heart disease. They may actually be more impressed with things that are of more immediate concern to them. Tobacco makes you smell and taste bad, which makes a pretty good argument with teens who are concerned about being attractive. (Although they can get around that one by finding a boyfriend or girlfriend who also smokes.) You may be able to reach kids who are physically active by explaining that smoking reduces stamina. It's hard to run the 440 when you're coughing your head off!

Drugs. Many prescription and over-the-counter drugs have effects that are important to consider in managing diabetes. For example, drugs may raise or lower blood glucose, affect heart rate, interfere with sexual function, or upset the stomach. If your child with diabetes takes a prescription or over-the-counter drug, ask your pharmacist if it has any diabetes-specific effects.

Illegal drugs. Recreational drugs—also called drugs of abuse—have many potential negative effects, only a few of which are specific to blood sugar control. Marijuana and cocaine, for example, affect the appetite, so they can influence diabetes management.

Marijuana is notorious for bringing on the "munchies," or eating binges. Just about anything edible seems to be fair game, but sweets are particularly attractive. Marijuana munchies can lead to pretty outrageous disturbances in diabetes control. Someone high on pot is probably not thinking clearly enough to calculate the supplemental insulin dose for a whole bag of chocolate chip cookies! In fact, one of the most profound ways in which all forms of substance abuse affects diabetes management relates to the altered states they produce. Being drunk or high usually leads to abandonment of basic self-care. The test doesn't get done. The meal gets skipped. The dose of insulin is forgotten or taken incorrectly.

Quite the opposite of marijuana, cocaine may reduce appetite and contribute to weight loss. This is, in fact, one of its attractions for some people. Cocaine acts like epinephrine, or adrenaline. Because of this, it may raise blood glucose in spite of the reduction in appetite and food intake it usually causes.

Of course, these and other drugs of abuse have many other negative effects. If you suspect your teen is using drugs, blood glucose control may be the least of your worries. We encourage you to get the information and support you and your child need to deal with this serious problem. Your pharmacist, physician, and diabetes educator are all good resources.

Sex. Most parents wish that teens would abstain from sex until they're older, but the fact is that many teens are sexually active. AIDS and other sexually transmitted diseases, as well as the risk of unwanted pregnancy, are just some of the dangers involved. Since unprotected sex with the wrong person could cost a teen his life in the era of AIDS, many realistic parents have seen to it that their child (boy or girl) has condoms—just in case.

Diabetes adds its own complications. Like any type of physical exertion, sex can produce low blood sugar. Risk for hypoglycemia during or after sexual intercourse is greater if blood sugar is on the low side to begin with and if insulin levels are fairly high. Prevention and treatment are the same as for any form of physical activity, but few teens will have the forethought and self-confidence to test blood sugar and stop for a snack before (or while) having sex. (Maybe there ought to be a tube of glucose gel with the condoms—just in case.)

Discuss the situation frankly with your teenager. If sexual activity is a possibility (or a reality), one of you needs to discuss contraceptive options with the healthcare team. Birth control pills are the most reliable form of contraception, and women with diabetes can use them. However, pills alone don't confer any protection against AIDS and other sexually transmitted diseases. The only truly safe option is abstinence, but proper condom use greatly reduces the risk for disease transmission when compared with unprotected sex. Next to abstinence, pills and condoms together provide the greatest possible protection against both pregnancy and sexually transmitted disease.

Another diabetes-specific risk of sex is pregnancy. Of course, teen pregnancy has huge implications for everyone concerned: the young mother and father, the baby, the grandparents, and the society as a whole. If the pregnant teen has diabetes, the problems and risks can be greatly multiplied. When pregnancy in diabetes is expertly managed, the health of the baby and the mother are no different than for any other pregnancy. However, diabetes control has to be excellent *before* conception as well as throughout the next nine months. In other words, the pregnancy must be planned—which is rarely the case when a teen becomes pregnant outside of marriage. If the mother's glucose control is not good when she conceives, the baby is at significant risk for birth defects.

The nutritional needs of a pregnant teen with diabetes are pretty high as well. Pregnancy alone increases the need for calories, protein, folic acid, iron, and several other nutrients. When those needs are superimposed on the high energy and nutrient demands created by teenage growth and development, the nutritional stakes get pretty high. Finally, add the complexity of balancing nutritional intake with insulin to produce stellar glucose control. Now you have a difficult situation on your hands. A pregnant teen with diabetes needs to work closely with a skilled dietitian or other diabetes educator to help her with this complex task. An endocrinologist (to help manage the diabetes) and an obstetrician/gynecologist (to follow the pregnancy) are also needed.

Helping Your Teen to Want Better Control

Blood sugar control during the teen years is a huge challenge. It takes a lot of hard work and perseverance at a time when most kids would certainly prefer to forget they even have diabetes. And since a teen doesn't get visible rewards out of better control, the chance of him doing all those hard self-care tasks is small, unless you can find the right motivator.

The risk of long-term complications just doesn't impress most teens, because they live in the here and now. Twenty years into the future doesn't seem real to them. Most adolescents also have a general feeling of invincibility—bad things may happen to other people but not to them. They may understand the risks intellectually but simply not feel personally vulnerable. Motivators, to be powerful, need to be personal and more immediate: perhaps things like feeling your best, being able to participate in sports, and avoiding hypoglycemia and the embarrassment and disruption it can cause.

One of the best arguments for better control that we have found—especially for boys—is that poor control places growth, both height and muscle mass, at risk. Most young men want to reach their full growth potential, to be strong, and to have good muscle mass—none of which can happen when diabetes control is poor. Reaching full height is also important to many girls. The shorter a person is, the lower her energy needs, and the fewer calories she burns, so she may need to be more careful about food intake and exercise all through her life in order to prevent unwanted weight gain.

Help your teen think through the benefits of better control. Every kid is different. He needs to be clear about what he wants. Lots of questions and discussion are the best approaches we know of to help him find the answers.

Pumps or Multiple Injections for Teens

Stringent blood glucose goals are not a realistic option for most teens because of their hormonal changes, rebelliousness, and irregular schedules. These challenges cause many diabetes programs to routinely exclude teens from intensive therapy—whether multiple injections, a pump, or insulin adjustments—yet many teens could benefit greatly from this approach, even if they are not trying for optimal control. These tools offer flexibility for adjusting food and insulin to meet actual demands and can also be a big help for teens who take part in sports or other activities that cause day-to-day variations in insulin demand. In other words, for just about any teenager.

To control glucose on standard insulin regimens, unchanging insulin doses must be paired with unchanging food and exercise, every day. Maintaining that kind of stability and self-discipline is hard for anyone, especially for a teen. So pumps, pens, and rapid-acting insulin can be particularly welcome to them.

Pumps provide the greatest flexibility because a person doesn't need to eat a certain amount at a given time. Teens can also reduce insulin during exercise—even when they didn't plan to be active—thus lowering the risk for low blood sugars during and after exercise. And they can sleep late on the weekend without having to take a morning shot.

But there is a downside to all that flexibility. The wearer must pay more attention to his diabetes, checking the infusion set every day, changing it every couple of days, and being doubly responsible about blood sugar testing. Many teens find it hard to deal with the pump's visibility. Depending on how the pump is worn, it can make diabetes more obvious—and a source of curiosity—to people around you. Some teens can't deal with someone else seeing it, whether in gym class, at the beach, or in more intimate moments. Some teens also object to the pump because it interferes with their body image, and the thought of being dependent on a machine may be disturbing in itself.

The issues of pump acceptance during the sensitive teen years seem to be much less of a factor for kids who began wearing a pump at a younger age. They already have the skill and know the benefits. The pump is just a fact of life.

Multiple injection therapy (MDI), preferably using a pen for ease and convenience, is another option for enhanced flexibility. It's not as precise as a pump, but with the right background insulin to allow flexible timing of meals and rapid-acting insulin instead of regular for meals, MDI can work very well.

The teen years with diabetes can be tough, and flexible therapy can help lighten the load. But selling that to your teen may not be easy. A form of therapy that requires more injections, tests, or other self-care tasks probably won't be a popular idea at first. But a frank discussion of the benefits can help.

Family Meals Are Still Important

Many teens want to eat all their meals away from home, but family mealtimes are still valuable. The more they eat at home, the better their overall nutrition will be, because kids are more likely to drink milk and eat fruits and vegetables at home than at other places. These foods provide important nutrients that tend to be missing from the diets of teens who seldom eat at home. And the benefits of family meals extend far beyond nutrition. With time together becoming more limited as your teen grows up, family meals are a great way to reconnect.

The parents' job description remains the same even though your teen is eating fewer meals with the family.

1. Get the right stuff into the house and onto the table. Teens eat a lot of snacks, and you can greatly improve the quality of what they eat by stocking healthy ones: fruits, bagels, whole-grain breads, lean meats and low-fat cheeses for sandwiches, low-fat or skim milk, yogurt, soup, and cereal. These foods contribute to good nutrition

and health while filling up that gaping, bottomless pit of teenage hunger. High-fat, high-sugar snack foods just fill the pit.

2. Continue to have family meals and expect the kids to be there, even though you know they won't always make it. This reinforces the message that regular meals are important. If teens can't be at a family meal because of other commitments, they should let you know. This shows respect for your efforts in preparing meals, and it keeps the teen hooked into the family process, even though he's not always participating in it actively.

THE BOTTOM LINE

1. The physical, developmental, and emotional upheavals of adolescence make diabetes control a real challenge. Somewhat less ambitious blood sugar goals may be needed.

2. Parents need to stay involved in the teen's diabetes and avoid criticizing his or her self-care efforts.

3. The teen's desire for privacy and the possible emergence of sensitive issues like sex and alcohol make this a good time to start independent doctor visits.

4. Teens' erratic schedules call for sophisticated management skills guided by the results of blood sugar testing.

5. Teens need early, accurate education about the effects and risks of alcohol use in diabetes.

6. The interaction of diabetes with driving, sex, and drugs needs frank discussion to keep your teen safe.

7. The tools of intensive therapy—multiple injections or a pump, and insulin adjustments for changes in food and activity—can add much-needed flexibility to a teen's management plan. These tools can be useful even with less demanding blood sugar goals.

13

An Action Plan for Avoiding "Diabetes Overwhelmus Mom-and-Popus"

When Dave and Lonnie came to the office, they were like most parents we are seeing for the first time: concerned, loving, tired, and overwhelmed. "We haven't been out together alone since our daughter Trudy developed diabetes," Dave told us. "Lonnie's afraid to leave her with a baby-sitter. She does every blood sugar check and insulin shot herself and makes every meal. She's the one who knows the most about it, so she takes care of it. Sometimes I feel like I've lost my wife, like I'm living with this really intense nurse."

"I just feel better doing it myself," Lonnie countered. "I wouldn't enjoy myself if we went out anyway. I'd be too worried that Trudy was home conning the sitter out of stuff she shouldn't eat or running around so much that she has a reaction or something."

The parents were suffering from a bad case of what we call diabetes overwhelmus mom-and-popus. Don't let the silly name fool you. This is a serious threat—and it spells trouble for the whole family.

Paying so much attention to diabetes can make you neglect yourself, your partner, and your relationship.

Lonnie and Dave were overwhelmed. Their own needs were buried under the weight of the daily management of Trudy's diabetes. Fun and relaxation were a thing of the past, and they were stressed and unhappy. Each of them felt frustrated and alone, and their marriage was suffering.

Trudy's control was quite good when we first saw her family, but all of them were paying a high price for it. And like most parents, they couldn't keep up this pace indefinitely. Eventually, the stress would lead to arguments and burnout. The family's quality of life and even its long-term survival were endangered.

Paying so much attention to diabetes can make you neglect yourself, your partner, and your relationship. Yet if there's one thing a child with diabetes needs, it's sane, healthy parents who are happy, relaxed, and secure. You are your child's advocate, protector, and role model. If you get exhausted and frustrated, she will feel the fallout in a negative way—even if you got that way doing things for her welfare!

Staying Sane and Healthy

Get the whole family involved. Regardless of how old your child is, you, the child, and everyone else in the family need to work together, as a team. Diabetes care is a partnership: a cooperative effort among all the members of the family.

Often, Mom ends up doing too much: going to all the medical appointments, taking responsibility for the food, giving all the injections and finger sticks, and so on. Dad has to be a part of this, too, taking an active role in the daily care. And other kids in the family, in age-appropriate ways, can help. Not only does this free up some of Mom's time to work on other family needs and on keeping her own balance and sanity, but it's also reassuring for the child with diabetes to feel that larger network of support around him. Dad and the kids will benefit from it too. Their help is really needed, and giving it will make them feel good.

Various techniques can help distribute the diabetes load. One is to break up routine care into individual tasks and then divide the tasks among family members. Another is to ask the child with diabetes what kind of help he wants from other family members.

Make sure that your blood sugar goals are realistic. Remember, perfect control is impossible to achieve using the medical tools we have available now. This is especially true during your child's teenage years, when emotional and hormonal changes can make blood sugar control particularly rocky. Cut your child and yourself a little slack. Agree on "good-enough" goals that keep the child feeling well and the self-care burden manageable. You will find it improves both your family life and your child's willingness to work at controlling her diabetes.

Get feelings out in the open. Diabetes makes life more stressful, so everyone in your family is bound to feel angry, frustrated, and even scared at times. These and other feelings are inevitable, and they can also really drag down your family's quality of life. That's why it is so important to find ways to deal with these feelings. First, recognize that diabetes is the source of these feelings, not each other. Make sure everyone in the family stays on the same side of the fence. A family united to deal with diabetes can get a lot more done than one that's constantly blaming each other.

Getting feelings out in the open is also important. We are not talking about *acting out* the feelings; we are talking about *acknowledging* them so you can figure out how to deal with them. If getting things out in the open hasn't been your family's style, you may wonder exactly how to go about it. The best way depends on the specific feeling in question and on your child's age and personality. Young kids often get relief (and a good laugh) when they unleash their anger at diabetes by stomping around the house yelling, "I hate diabetes!" You might find it helpful too. Feel free to join the parade. Your kid will love it that you're being a little silly and that you feel the same as she does. Punching pillows or throwing them against a blank wall is another popular way to vent. (Be careful about throwing a pillow into a corner and kicking it hard. We know of one dad who broke a big toe when he got carried away during an I Hate Diabetes Parade.) Less physical youngsters may prefer drawing angry pictures—smashed syringes, dismantled blood test meters, and the like. Older kids sometimes get relief from simply talking about their hurt, anger, or resentment.

Why kids should express their "negative" feelings. Painful as it may be for you to hear your child express her sad or angry feelings, it's important to let her do it. Pain is a fact of life. It's not unique to diabetes, but diabetes definitely adds to the load. Parents sometimes feel they can lessen the pain by telling their children that diabetes isn't really so bad, that the child shouldn't feel as she does. In our experience, this only makes matters worse. The child knows how she feels. The parent's efforts to get her to feel otherwise almost always backfire, making her feel bad about herself or feel cut off from her parents, or both.

Feeling bad about diabetes is natural and normal, maybe even inevitable. When your child expresses these feelings and you acknowledge them, they become less of a problem. Parents can feel powerless when their child talks about how much she hates diabetes, because they don't know what to do about those feelings. They think they should be able to make the pain go away, even though they know this is not possible. Feelings need to be expressed, accepted, and dealt with. The most helpful thing you can do is to listen to your child with love.

How about *your* feelings? What should you do when you are frustrated, angry, and scared about things your child has done or not done about her diabetes care? You, too, need to let those feelings out. The key to doing this constructively is to talk about how you are feeling, not about what your child is doing. If, for example, your child is having a tough time staying away from some food that sends her blood sugar through the roof, you may be tempted to blame her for "cheating." But blaming won't change her behavior, and it's almost guaranteed to drive a wedge between you. Instead, try telling her how her behavior makes you feel: scared, frustrated, or confused.

This approach probably won't get your child to immediately go back on her nutrition plan. But you will have found a way to vent your feelings without driving her away. This will help prevent excess anger and resentment from building up over time.

It takes practice to become good at expressing feelings instead of blaming, so it's possible (especially at first) that your child may respond by feeling as if you were criticizing her. If this happens, you can tell her that you are not blaming her; though you wish you could control her behavior, you know you can't. This not only is a valuable release for you, it also models for the child effective ways to deal with her own angry or hurt feelings.

Obviously, the extent to which you share your feelings with your child depends on how old she is. This technique probably is not much use with very young children, though sharing feelings of anger at the diabetes or resentment at the demands and restrictions it imposes works with kids of any age.

Healthcare Is a Team Effort

Know what's needed medically and ask for it—if necessary, demand it.
The American Diabetes Association and others have defined good diabetes care. An excellent way to deal with the fears you have about your child's health is to know what the experts say needs to be done and then double check that your own team is following through.

Minimum care includes a doctor's visit at least four times a year, to see a nurse, dietitian, and counselor (if available) and to check:

- weight, height, and blood pressure
- A1C levels
- blood lipids, kidney function, and eyes (once each year)

These visits will enable you to:

- Ensure that growth and development are normal
- Get a long-term sense of blood sugar control
- Adjust treatment to keep pace with changes in child's body and life
- Monitor for potential problems
- Keep your diabetes management skills current
- Help your child take steps toward controlling her own diabetes.

Build a good relationship with your child's diabetes healthcare team. Your child's healthcare team is extremely important to your confidence and success in dealing with diabetes. Your doctor and educators have important knowledge and skills to share with you, but you need a good relationship with them to benefit. If you have communication problems with the team or philosophical differences about diabetes management, they won't be able to meet your needs.

Every doctor treating a child with diabetes should be aware of appropriate standards of care (*see bulleted items above*) and should provide the necessary services. And because food is so important, make sure your team includes a dietitian who knows kids and diabetes. If it doesn't, ask your doctor for a referral.

Different families want different types of relationships with their teams. Some need a lot of guidance—when a child is newly diagnosed or is going through a particularly difficult time, for example. Others prefer to be independent, with their team acting more as advisers.

Do your part to ensure that you get what you need from your team. Be prepared for appointments by jotting down questions or problems in advance. Listen carefully to the answers. Take notes or ask for a written copy of any instructions or information. Don't be afraid to speak up when you don't understand. No doctor or educator can answer every question, but they should be willing to find out the answer. They may not know exactly what it's like to live with diabetes, but they should be accepting and compassionate.

If you're not getting what you need, speak up. Talking through any difficulties is the first step to solving them. How your doctor and team respond to your concerns and questions will tell you whether the relationship can work for you. Changing doctors shouldn't be taken lightly, however, and if your health coverage is obtained through a managed care plan, it may not even be an option. But if the relationship isn't working, talk to your doctor or your insurance company representative about what you can do. The right healthcare team is an immeasurable help.

Take Care of Your Inner Self

Give yourself credit for trying; mistakes are a part of learning. All learning requires us to try new things. And trying something new means that we will make mistakes.

It's been said that you have to be willing to do something badly in order to learn to do it well. That certainly is true of diabetes care. So try to use the mistakes to help you learn—high blood sugar readings, for example, can be seen as a clue in a detective story instead of a failure that leaves you feeling frustrated and beaten. And while you're learning, give yourself and your child credit for trying. A pat on the back, a hug, or a cheer can put the failures in perspective and keep the learning process going.

Laurie, one mother we worked with, felt like a failure after trying the new, more liberal approach to sweets. A dietitian at a lecture described a study in which chocolate cake was substituted for other carbohydrate in the diets of people with diabetes without impairing blood sugar control. This was great news for Laurie, because the thing her son Cody missed most since his diabetes had been diagnosed was the great milk-chocolate cake from a neighborhood bakery. Laurie bought one of the cakes on the way home, and Cody had a nice big piece after dinner. But either the lecturer had left out some important part of the puzzle or Cody's overall situation wasn't conducive to a piece of cake that night, because his bedtime blood sugar was 312 mg/dl (17.4 mmol).

"I should have known it was too good to be true," she moaned. "Now I'll have to throw out the cake and tell Cody it was a mistake." With a little discussion, however, we were able to redefine the episode as a learning opportunity and help Laurie cut herself a little slack. That first experiment with sweets wasn't a failure, because it had shown them what didn't work for Cody. It was the first step in figuring out what *does* work. And Mom needed credit for going to the lecture to learn more about diabetes and for caring enough to try something that Cody would enjoy so much.

The story of Thomas Edison and the light bulb illustrates how we need to look at diabetes self-care experiments that don't work out. Edison conducted over 5,000 experiments without succeeding in developing a light bulb that worked. One day, a reporter asked why he didn't give up; how could he stand to fail 5,000 times? Edison replied, "I haven't failed once; I'm 5,000 steps closer to the solution!"

Don't accept guilt, whether from healthcare workers, family, or friends, and watch out for the "diabetes police." Have you ever been busted by the "diabetes police"? The diabetes police, or DPs, are people who offer unsolicited comments or advice about what you or your child are doing. They come in many varieties: perfectionist healthcare providers, nosy neighbors, gloating grandmas, and frank friends. They mean well. Their knowledge base may even be excellent ("You should have given at least three extra units for that muffin—they have over 50 grams of carbohydrate each, you know!") or awful ("I just couldn't give my child shots every day. I heard if you gave them chromium supplements, they wouldn't need those terrible shots.") Whether their comments are helpful, hurtful, or just plain stupid, they assume you're doing something wrong or that you're ignorant of some crucial fact about diabetes care. And if you're already feeling uncertain or frustrated, these comments can send you over the edge.

How do you cope? Some parents tell us they just run a little tape in their heads: "He means well, but he doesn't know what he's talking about. We're doing the right thing." Others may respond out loud: "I appreciate your concern, Mom, but we've discussed this with Jason's doctor. These foods are fine for his diabetes." Some let their DPs know exactly how they feel about the comments: "I get a little defensive when you make comments like that, Dad. We all work hard to take care of Troy's diabetes. It would help me a lot if you would ask us what's going on when you're concerned, instead of trying to give us advice."

Perfectionist providers. Perhaps the hardest DPs to deal with are the perfectionist doctors and other healthcare providers who have impossible expectations. These misguided souls tend to berate you when your management of diabetes is less than perfect. In response, you might point out how few people in the DCCT intensive treatment group ever achieved normal blood sugars. Even with the best of care and support, only about 20 percent ever achieved a normal A1C during the whole nine years. Only about five percent of the group was able to keep it normal. Tell them also that you're working hard to get the best control possible. You might add that you sometimes feel pressured by their standards, which makes it difficult for you and your child to do your best.

Your answers will vary, depending on the source and the content of the comment. But however you respond, don't accept the guilt. You don't deserve it, and it's not helpful.

Build an effective support system for yourself and your child. Diabetes is sometimes too much one person, or even one family, to handle alone. When this happens, get help. Some people hesitate to ask for help because they feel it would be a burden or an imposition, but most people who care about you and your child are willing to do whatever they can to help. In fact, they are likely to feel flattered by your confidence in them and certainly will feel closer to you as a result of the shared task of keeping the family well.

Sources of support. Friends and relatives can be a vital support network. For many families, they are the best source of the kind of loving childcare that will allow Mom and Dad some relatively worry-free personal time, away from the demands of diabetes.

Support groups for parents are another great resource and can help you with the many practical and other issues related to diabetes. The American Diabetes Association or Juvenile Diabetes Foundation chapters in your area as well as some hospitals and other organizations may provide such services. You could also consider turning to a trusted minister, rabbi, or other spiritual leader for support, advice, or a shoulder to cry on.

And don't forget the support to your mental health that comes from hobbies and other activities. Make time for whatever gives you joy and relaxes you. You'll have more to give and a better attitude as a result.

Diabetes is a big load. Don't hesitate to reach out to others for help. Remember though, to give back. Helping others when you can—in the family, the community, or parent support groups—is part of what makes the system work. This give and take helps everyone to get what she needs without feeling as if she is being taken advantage of.

Give Yourself a Break

Take regular breaks from the diabetes by yourself and as a couple (or with other friends and family if you're a single parent). One of the most important functions of a support system for parents is that it enables you to take a break. We've found that for many families, it takes at least a year after the diagnosis to start living normally again. Each family has its own definition of "normal," of course. Parents who were active and had a booming social life before diabetes need to find a way to get back in the swing of things. But if your idea of a big night is renting a movie and munching popcorn with the kids, nestled in a big comforter in front of the TV, you may not have as much adjusting to do.

Some parents have a hard time leaving their child with diabetes with another caregiver. They are afraid something will go wrong in their absence. It seems that the younger the child is at diagnosis, the more difficult this is. If you are having this problem, find a way to overcome it, for your own good, the good of your marriage, and that of your child. Train the baby-sitter or grandma. Make the first outings short and close to home to build your confidence gradually. And, if necessary, get a beeper or cell phone so you can be reached in an emergency. Do whatever it takes to get some time for yourself and for your relationship, free of the worries and demands of diabetes.

Your child with diabetes needs you happy and healthy. If you crash and burn, her most important teacher, advocate, and support is gone. If you won't take time for yourself for your own needs, do it for the sake of your child.

Protect your own physical health through good eating, enjoyable activities, and frequent laughter. Your body needs care, too. Take time to do the things for your own health that you want your child to do for hers. Managing diabetes is no job for weaklings. You need your strength—physical as well as mental—to cope. Eating well is one important part of a healthy lifestyle that will keep you feeling your best. Get enough sleep and a reasonable amount of physical activity every day. Individual preference, personality, and fitness level all affect the type and amount of activity that are best for you.

Any kind of aerobic activity—walking, jogging, bike riding, gardening, dancing, baseball, doubles tennis, in-line skating—keeps the heart healthy, improves circulation, increases strength and endurance, and reduces tension. And remember—kids raised in a physically active family are more likely to be active as teenagers and adults.

And while you're out there jogging around the block and eating your vegetables, have a good laugh now and then. It tones up muscles, lowers blood pressure, improves the immune response, and makes you feel wonderful!

THE BOTTOM LINE

1. To help your child grow up healthy, you must stay on an even keel yourself. Otherwise, the demands of diabetes on top of normal daily stresses may overwhelm you.
2. To maintain your own health and sanity, involve the whole family (and close friends) in living with diabetes. Give everyone a chance to help out.
3. Make sure your blood sugar goals for your child are realistic; trying to be perfect is a recipe for disaster.
4. Build a strong relationship with your child's diabetes healthcare providers and be sure she is getting the care she needs and deserves.
5. Take care of yourself: Eat well, get enough rest, spend time with people you love, do things you enjoy, and laugh as often as possible.

14

Helping Your Child Learn to Live with Diabetes

Russ was 20, and after two years at the local junior college, he decided the time had come for him to leave for college. He wanted to be an architect, and the design school was some 400 miles from home, in southern California. As the day of departure approached, he and his mother started to panic—they were both convinced that she was the only thing standing between the young man and utter disaster. Unlike most of the teenagers we see, Russ hadn't rebelled much against his mom's control of his diabetes. With few exceptions, he had kept a pretty regular schedule, carefully counted his carbohydrate, tested fairly often, and reviewed the numbers with his mom.

Mom was an extremely accomplished caregiver. Her skillful adjustments of insulin and activity had kept Russ's diabetes on an even keel for years. She managed diabetes during illness better than some endocrine resident physicians.

Both Russ and his mother were convinced that she was the only thing standing between the young man and utter disaster.

Unfortunately, she had neglected, out of love and concern, to help Russ learn to control his own blood sugars. So, here he was, at age 20, getting the short course in independent diabetes self-management. But without much time to practice those skills in a safe environment, he was heading off to college unprepared. And Mom was having trouble letting go. The only thing keeping her from moving to Los Angeles with her son ("just for the first semester or two, until I'm sure he's okay") was Dad's refusal to pay for two apartments there.

Who manages your child's diabetes? As you are well aware, diabetes care isn't managed by healthcare providers. It's controlled at home, at the soccer game, in school. With diabetes, success depends a lot less on the doctor's skill in picking the right therapy than it does on the ability of the child and the family to put that therapy to work in the real world. And by taking small steps at first and progressively larger ones as he grows into an independent adult, the child gradually develops the confidence and skills to make all those daily decisions to safely manage his own diabetes.

Your job/your child's job. If you keep in mind that your job is to help your child learn to control his blood sugars and not to control them yourself, you'll appreciate the benefits of helping him learn what works for his diabetes and his life. He probably wants to be as free of his diabetes as possible, and that's understandable. He wants to do the things other kids do. He wants to enjoy birthday parties, sleep over at friends' houses, and be as unencumbered by his diabetes as he can be. These are normal and achievable goals, and you can help him reach them. Doing your part means sympathizing with him when he's upset, helping him solve problems when he's stuck, praising him as often as possible, criticizing him as infrequently as possible, and loving him all the time.

Helping your child learn self-control means being clear about the difference between pushing and supporting. Everyone likes support, but no one likes to be pushed. When you support your child, you are helping him reach a goal he has chosen; when you push him, you are trying to get him to do something you have chosen. And he will probably resist. Your child shouldn't necessarily make diabetes management decisions on his own, but you should let him take the lead in making these decisions. You will be there to keep him out of trouble as he does this, to be sure, but you are giving him the chance to safely practice the skills he will need for the rest of his life.

Letting go is hard to do. This approach can be hard for parents. They fear their child will not do the right thing when it comes to diabetes care. And she might not, all of the time. But she'll do fine most of the time, if you work together, gradually shifting responsibility to her. If your child doesn't buy into the diabetes care plan you have laid out, she will find a way to undermine it anyway, so helping her learn to choose her own plan and make her own decisions is really the only way to go.

In the meantime, you might keep in mind the words of the serenity prayer: "God grant me the serenity to accept the things I cannot change, the courage to change the things I can, and the wisdom to know the difference." When you live by this credo, you are doing your part to help your child live a healthy life while keeping the bond between you strong.

Your child and his diabetes are unique. There are no cookbooks for diabetes management or for your child's development. You have to develop your own recipe. This means first learning the theory and techniques through reading books, taking classes, working with a diabetes educator, and going to support groups, for example. Then, using the techniques in this chapter, engage your child in his own care by passing on your skills in a safe environment.

Helping Him to Help Himself

Parenting Techniques

Ask questions. Questions are the most powerful tool you have for helping your child grow up healthy and happy. They're also terrific for preserving the peace. Asking questions is the foundation for your parent-child partnership in diabetes care, an essential strategy for safely passing on skills and responsibility to your child. (*See Chapter 5 for more on this subject.*)

You might ask such questions as, "What's the hardest thing for you right now about managing your diabetes?" "Is there anything I can do to help?" or "What do you think we should do about this situation?" All of these questions are open-ended invitations to your child to share his thoughts and participate in solving the problem.

Tone and timing are critical. When it comes to good questions, tone and timing are crucial. We're reminded of Tiffany, a 12-year-old who would never test her blood before dinner without a major hassle. Mom said she'd tried everything: getting the testing supplies and sitting with Tiffany, trying to force her to do the test, refusing to give her daughter dinner until she had done the test, and punishing her for not doing the test; all to no avail. Tiffany agreed that the situation was awful.

When the nurse asked Tiffany if she thought testing her blood before dinner was important, Tiffany said yes. She was at a loss, though, to explain exactly why she didn't do it. She didn't like interrupting what she was doing, she admitted, and she really hated having her mother tell her what to do. All the same, she acknowledged that she would probably not test on her own. It seemed there was no way out. Still, the nurse asked Tiffany if she could think of any way for her mother to help her test. After a little thought, Tiffany suggested an experiment: If her mother would ask her 10 minutes before dinner if she had tested, she would try to follow through.

At their next clinic appointment, Tiffany's mother declared, "Well, that idea certainly didn't work!" She had forgotten to remind Tiffany to test for the first few days after their last visit. She finally remembered on the fourth day, after dinner had already begun. At that point, she turned to Tiffany and said, "You didn't test, did you?!" Tone and timing—Tiffany's mom missed on both counts. Instead of being a supportive reminder, the question came out as an attack.

She had asked what we sometimes call a rhetorical question, one to which she already knew (or thought she knew) the answer. Another example of a rhetorical question is, "Did you eat those cookies that were on the counter?" when your child has high blood sugar and chocolate crumbs on his T-shirt.

When you ask questions, make them real ones. Ask questions designed to open up communication with your child, to give you information, and to help him take better care of himself. Avoid questions designed to blame or to catch your child making mistakes of judgment or behavior. Rhetorical questions only make matters worse; real questions attempt to find solutions to problems.

Learn from success too. When a problem situation goes more smoothly than usual, one of the most useful questions you can ask is "How come that worked so well?" Let's say your child usually finds it hard to limit himself to the amount that's been planned for his afternoon snack. Then one day he's fine with what you give him. Understanding what made the difference gives both of you important information. Maybe this particular snack was more filling, maybe he was less hungry than usual, or maybe he just ate his snack earlier than normal. By figuring out why things went well, you help your child identify effective strategies for controlling his diabetes. And focusing on successes rather than failures is the best way to learn.

Individualize. The best plan for managing diabetes is one that takes into account the unique individuals involved. Some kids really like routines, others hate them. Some children have no problem eating what's provided in the amounts offered, others can't live with the limits of set meal plans, and still others are such picky eaters that their parents live in constant dread of hypoglycemia. Some kids are totally at ease managing their diabetes in public, eating snacks, taking shots, and doing tests, no matter who notices. Others don't want people to know about their diabetes, and they wouldn't dream of taking a shot or doing a blood test in front of anyone. Some children feel their diabetes is an almost overwhelming burden, while others brush it off as a minor inconvenience.

And the aspect of diabetes that's most bothersome varies, as well. For one child it might be shots; for another, it's doctor's appointments or blood tests, not being able to eat as much candy as her friends, or having to stop during ball games for a snack. The list of potential individual differences is endless, but try to identify and work on the diabetes-related issues that cause the most stress in your family. Acknowledging your child's individual preferences and finding ways to work around them, whenever possible, works better than forcing her to adapt to a rigid style that doesn't suit her.

Individualize your goals as well. (*See Chapter 5 for more about picking "good enough" blood sugar goals.*) When you are working toward those goals, keep in mind that some kids simply have an easier time hitting target blood sugars than other kids do. Those who are have just recently been diagnosed are probably still in the "honeymoon" phase of their diabetes, when the pancreas is still producing some insulin. This can make blood sugars much easier to control than they will be later, after the last of the body's insulin disappears.

Children whose daily routines of eating, exercise, insulin administration, and sleeping are fairly predictable tend to have an easier time controlling blood sugars. And some kids' relative ease in achieving good blood sugar control can't be explained. Whatever the reason, if your child seems to get the blood sugar numbers you're all aiming for without much effort, your individual goals can be a bit more ambitious than if his diabetes were more difficult to manage.

Unfortunately, most kids don't have such an easy time of it. If your child is a teenager, is less given to routines, or has trouble easily achieving blood sugar control for any reason, you should adjust your goals accordingly. These goals should still be ambitious, to be sure, but they must also be realistic. Otherwise, you and your child will end up miserable and discouraged, making control even harder to achieve.

Be specific. As you work with your child toward your common goals, it's helpful if you can identify specific problems, vulnerabilities, strengths, and successes. Rita was a high school senior. She had been diagnosed with diabetes at the age of seven and had managed it well. Suddenly, she started running really high blood sugars. In fact, she was so hyperglycemic many mornings that she couldn't even drag herself out of bed to go to school. It turned out that Rita had been going to the mall every night after dinner and hanging out with her friends. One of their favorite activities, other than talking, was eating. Rita joined in, and by the time she got home, her blood sugar would be sky high. For some reason, Rita would tell herself that it was "too late" to do anything about the hyperglycemia at this point, and would just go to bed. As a result, she was up half the night urinating and was in big trouble the next morning. But by acknowledging and specifically describing the problem, she helped find a solution.

Naturally, the solution had to be equally specific, and Rita was very clear about some potential solutions that would not work for her. She would not 1) stop going to the mall, 2) stop eating when she went to the mall, 3) carry all her insulin paraphernalia with her to the mall, or 4) take an extra shot when she got home. Though in a way Rita was being difficult, her frankness made it crystal clear what would not work. The physician to whom Rita described her problem appreciated her honesty, and he racked his brains to come up with a solution. After offering a few suggestions that she vetoed, he came up with one she would try: carrying an insulin pen containing rapid-acing insulin to the mall in her purse. Rita said she would go to the bathroom right before she ate and give herself the right amount of insulin to cover the food she had ordered. This worked for her because she could do it quickly and discreetly.

As you work toward specific solutions with your child, keep this image in mind: If you can help your child describe a problem (or a solution) so specifically that you could make a movie of it, you are on the right track. Getting that specific takes time and work. It helps to ask probing questions and try to discover what's really going on, as if you were solving a mystery. Think about the energy that your child is willing to invest in things that really interest him (like getting some girl to notice him, for example). Wouldn't it be wonderful if he could tap that same energy and curiosity when learning to manage his diabetes?

Solving specific problems also helps people feel less overwhelmed. They are relieved to find that their sticking point is a particular piece of the regimen, rather than the whole thing. It makes living with diabetes feel more manageable.

Take a step-by-step approach. Any problem is easier to solve when you break it down into manageable steps. Diabetes-related problems are no exception. Think of any situation that you want to work on: helping your child begin doing his own shots, for example. Then think of all the steps involved in actually completing that task: getting out the insulin, choosing a pen needle, deciding how much insulin to give (if you are adjusting doses), priming the pen, dialing the dose, checking it, giving the shot, noting the amount of insulin given, and, finally, putting everything back where it belongs and disposing of the needle.

Once you've listed the steps, tell your child he can pick one step to do himself. (Make sure it's one that he can handle or that you can closely monitor.) Once he is comfortable taking responsibility for this first task (which may take a few days or even weeks), he can take on another. In this way, you help him learn the skills he needs to master one step at a time, with you there to make sure he is doing things right. This allows you to shift responsibility to your child gradually, so it's easier for him to manage. Almost any diabetes task can be broken down into steps and taught in this way.

This approach to helping your child learn diabetes self-control also lets you stay in touch with an older child, increasing the likelihood that nothing important will slip between the cracks. Stefan, whom you met in the introduction, has been using an insulin pump since he was 11 years old. When he was 20, just before he moved out on his own, his dad was still helping him change the insulin pump infusion set and refill the syringe. Stefan didn't really need the help, but it gave his Dad a chance to check on how things were going with his diabetes, and it was something they could share.

A gradual approach to responsibility for diabetes care builds confidence, facilitates independence, ensures that diabetes management tasks are attended to, and strengthens the parent-child relationship, all at the same time.

Here's one more tip for making the step-by-step technique work for your family. As you begin to divide up responsibilities for a task, don't just check up on your child; have him check up on you, too. Let him verify that you have drawn up the right amount of insulin, chosen acceptable foods for his lunch, or taken everything you need for your trip to the park. This approach shows the cooperative nature of diabetes care and helps your child begin to learn what he needs to know with a minimum of pressure.

Check regularly to see how things are going. Keeping on top of diabetes takes maintenance, so it's important to check in regularly with your child to see how she feels things are going. Ask her about any new problems that might have come up, about any successes she's had managing her diabetes, and about anything else you need to discuss. Some families have diabetes meetings regularly, where everyone gets to say whatever they want about how things have been going. This is a good chance to deal with small problems before they become big ones. The key to success with these meetings is maintaining an attitude of cooperation.

Maintaining contact is especially important as your child gets older and assumes more of the day-to-day management of her diabetes. Some aspects of the regimen can go undone if you give them up before your child is fully prepared to take them on, so regular contact and continued involvement can prevent trouble.

Keep in touch with other adults who regularly interact with your child, such as teachers, coaches, and youth-group leaders. Naturally, your child will want to know when you speak to these folks, and she might even want to be with you when you do. As we discussed earlier, these adults need to be well versed in managing potential diabetes-related emergencies, of which hypoglycemia is the most obvious example. Then check in occasionally to see if any problems have come up that you need to know about. (*See Chapter 11 about ensuring your child is well cared for at school.*)

Support problem-solving skills. We want our children to know they can do anything they set their minds to, as long as they can do it safely. One young man, Oliver, personifies effective diabetes problem solving. At the age of 11, just a few days after he got his first insulin pump, his dad took him to visit a friend in New York City. The friend didn't cook, so dinner at a local restaurant was planned. Oliver talked his father into letting him order anything he wanted—it was, after all, a special occasion— but when Oliver tested his blood just before ordering, his meter read 350 mg/dl (19 mmol). Dad knew the boy wanted to order dessert too, and images of a midnight visit to the emergency room flashed through his mind. It would have been understandable if Dad had followed his first instinct to go back on his agreement. But he didn't.

Instead, he decided to take a chance on his son's budding diabetes problem-solving skills, and maybe even strengthen them in the process. Dad said he would stick with the agreement on the condition that Oliver think really hard about how much insulin he needed to take, and that he test his blood two hours and four hours after dinner.

Oliver readily agreed and then proceeded to eat a big dinner, followed by coconut custard pie à la mode. Two hours later, his blood sugar was 220 mg/dl (12.2 mmol), and four hours later, it was 140 mg/dl (7.8 mmol). Oliver and his dad were both delighted, of course. When asked how he had managed to figure out how much insulin he needed to cover the meal, Oliver explained that he'd used the formula he'd been taught to calculate the insulin dose based on the amount of carbohydrate eaten. "I really wanted that food, Dad, but I didn't want to feel sick later, so I was extra careful when I counted it. Working hard like that is worth it when I can see I got the insulin right!"

Ask questions as part of the problem-solving process. How can you safely do that thing you've got your heart set on? If something goes wrong, remember to give credit for the effort, and then ask questions to learn as much as possible from the experience. You'll have a better starting point the next time a similar situation arises. And if it goes well, try to find out why so you can learn from that experience, too.

Get Help If You Need It

Teaching children to control blood sugars is difficult, and sometimes it can be overwhelming. You may need a professional to help you figure out what is going on and how to make things right. If your child is suffering from a psychological problem like depression (which is more common when kids have diabetes), counseling and medication can help. If your child is having trouble coping with the daily demands of diabetes, turn to his healthcare team for assistance. Working together, you can help your child build his confidence and skills.

Cultivate Emotional Strength

Dealing effectively with diabetes requires emotional strength as well as problem-solving skills. We've found that the fundamental elements of this emotional strength are love, faith, and humor. If you can foster these qualities in yourself and nurture them in your child, you will do well in your lives with diabetes.

Love. Make sure the hassles and aggravations of daily life with diabetes don't prevent you from enjoying, appreciating, and loving your child as fully as you can. One nine-year-old we know went through a period when he decided that his shots would hurt less if he did them slowly. Often, his mother would sit with him in the morning for five minutes or more as he—slowly, very slowly—pressed the needle to his skin. The performance was hard for her to bear, and the need to get him to school on time made it even worse. She wisely kept her frustration to herself, but one day she reached her limit.

"I know those shots must really hurt," she said. "Even just watching you, I get a knot in my stomach. I love you so much, if I could take half your shots for you, I would." Her son looked at her quizzically for a moment. Then he responded, "It doesn't hurt that much, Mom," and he pushed the needle right in. Turns out all he needed was that little boost that came from knowing he was loved. In fact, he never went back to his slow-motion injection method.

Faith and hope. Faith is another bulwark against the stresses and strains of daily life with diabetes. If you and your child have faith in a higher power, you can draw on the strength it provides you. And other kinds of faith can help as well: faith in modern medical technology, in your diabetes healthcare team, and in yourselves. One woman we know was diagnosed with diabetes over 40 years ago. No one in her family had ever had diabetes before, so it was unknown territory for all of them. Yet when the girl asked her mother what having diabetes would mean for them, her mom told her, "It means we will learn to eat better than we have ever eaten before, and we will all be healthier than we ever were before, and we will all learn to love each other more than we ever did before." Now, that's faith!

One 11-year-old was sitting with his father talking about wishes. When his father said he wished his son didn't have diabetes, the boy said, "I don't wish that. Not that I like diabetes; in fact, I hate it. But having diabetes has forced me to learn how to take care of myself. I can take care of myself better than any of my friends, and I wouldn't give that up for anything."

When we succeed in helping our children have faith in themselves, we are giving them one of life's most precious gifts. It will help them live well with their diabetes and with all the other challenges they will face in life. Naturally, to help your child have faith, you must have it yourself. Think of the things that buoy you up. Think of the things from which you draw strength and inspiration. If you have trouble doing this, try the following exercise.

For a few days, before you go to sleep each night, remind yourself of three things you did that day to help your child live a better life with diabetes. Then remind yourself of three things your child did to work toward the same goal. All too often, we lose sight of our accomplishments and successes. Bringing them to mind can help keep us strong and build our confidence.

Humor. How often have you heard someone say, "I don't know how I would have made it if it hadn't been for my sense of humor"? You may have even said it yourself. Humor helps you put things in perspective and can keep you from feeling overwhelmed. And you can help your child use humor to cope with his life with diabetes. Many years ago, when Mark was first diagnosed at the age of 10, he was given just one shot each morning, but soon his physician recommended adding a second shot at dinnertime. Mark didn't like this at all, and he pitched a fit every night, demanding to know why he couldn't go on taking just one shot a day. For several weeks his mother explained, over and over and in ever-increasing detail, the benefits of that second shot. All to no avail.

Finally, when Mark asked again one night, "Why can't I take just one shot a day?" she responded, "I can't think of a single reason. But why stop with one shot a day, why can't you take just one shot a week?" Getting into the swing of things, her son suggested one shot a month, and his mother retorted, "Let's go for the whole ball of wax: one shot a year!" Laughing, the boy said, "But think about how big the syringe would have to be!" Being good in math, he calculated that it would have to hold 12,775 units of insulin—that's one heck of a syringe!

The boy took his evening shot from then on without a fuss. Apparently, the shot had not been the real problem at all—it was just the last straw. It marked the point at which the boy went from barely being able to cope with having diabetes to being overwhelmed by it. The boy was really saying, "I'm overwhelmed. Help me lighten the load." Humor can do that, and it did.

Sometimes, it's the child who puts the situation into perspective. When she was seven, Julia went on a camping trip with her parents to a beautiful but isolated area. Unfortunately, on the second day of their vacation, a huge storm struck, drenching their tent and everything in it, including them. To make matters worse, at the height of the storm Julia's blood sugar fell so low that she could not swallow anything, and her parents had to give her a shot of glucagon, which they had wisely packed. The glucagon revived her, but as they tried to feed her to keep her blood sugar up, she began to vomit. And she vomited and vomited. For hours she sat there, soaking wet, with her head in a bucket. Her parents, equally wet, were pretty miserable as well. Finally, as Julia leaned over the bucket yet again, she lifted her head, smiled wanly, and said, "Oh, bad day . . ." At this, her parents started to laugh. Julia quickly joined in, and soon they were all feeling a lot better.

The essence of humor is taking a bad situation and exaggerating its awfulness to the point where it's so ridiculous it becomes funny. For better or for worse, life with diabetes presents us with plenty of material for humor. Try to find some in your daily life and see what you can make of it.

Eyes on the Prize

Managing food and nutrition is just a part of the overall picture of a well-functioning family. When you do your job—getting the right food on the table and, in a more general way, helping your child with diabetes learn to control his own blood sugars—you have met the bigger challenge. Remember your goal: a happy, healthy, independent child. When you continue to love and support him and stay involved with his diabetes as he grows to young adulthood, you are helping him to be strong, confident, and open to new challenges—now and for the rest of his life.

THE BOTTOM LINE

1. Your most important job is to help your child learn to control his own diabetes. Kids are never too young to begin taking part in their own care, and they are never too old to benefit from some support from their parents. Start working cooperatively when your child is young, and stay involved through the teen years.
2. Asking good questions is the most powerful tool you have for helping your child learn to control his own blood sugars.
3. Everyone learns best from successes, so focus on what your child does right rather than what he does wrong.
4. Each child is unique. Help your child develop specific, step-by-step approaches to the problems that bother him most.
5. Get help when you need it to protect your child from psychological problems and to strengthen your skills and resources for dealing with the daily demands of diabetes.
6. Emotional strength, based on love, faith, and humor, is fundamental for living well with diabetes. Foster these qualities in yourself, and nurture them in your child.

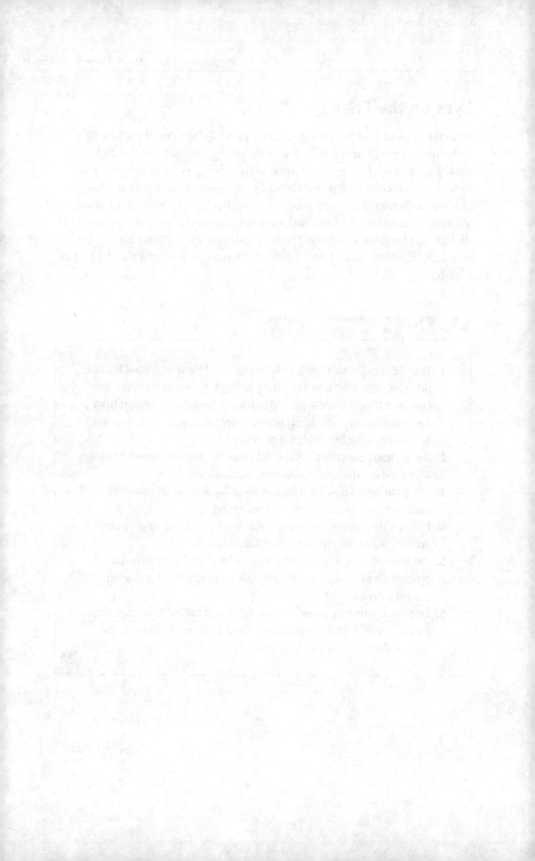

Index

About the American Diabetes Association

The American Diabetes Association is the nation's leading voluntary health organization supporting diabetes research, information, and advocacy. Its mission is to prevent and cure diabetes and to improve the lives of all people affected by diabetes. The American Diabetes Association is the leading publisher of comprehensive diabetes information. Its huge library of practical and authoritative books for people with diabetes covers every aspect of self-care— cooking and nutrition, fitness, weight control, medications, complications, emotional issues, and general self-care.

To order American Diabetes Association books: Call 1-800-232-6733. Or log on to http://store.diabetes.org

To join the American Diabetes Association: Call 1-800-806-7801. www.diabetes.org/membership

For more information about diabetes or ADA programs and services: Call 1-800-342-2383. E-mail: Customerservice@diabetes.org or log on to www.diabetes.org

To locate an ADA/NCQA Recognized Provider of quality diabetes care in your area: Call 1-703-549-1500 ext. 2202. www.diabetes.org/recognition/Physicians/ListAll.asp

To find an ADA Recognized Education Program in your area: Call 1-888-232-0822. www.diabetes.org/recognition/education.asp

To join the fight to increase funding for diabetes research, end discrimination, and improve insurance coverage: Call 1-800-342-2383. www.diabetes.org/advocacy

To find out how you can get involved with the programs in your community: Call 1-800-342-2383. See below for program Web addresses.

- *American Diabetes Month:* Educational activities aimed at those diagnosed with diabetes—month of November. www.diabetes.org/ADM
- *American Diabetes Alert:* Annual public awareness campaign to find the undiagnosed—held the fourth Tuesday in March. www.diabetes.org/alert
- *The Diabetes Assistance & Resources Program (DAR):* diabetes awareness program targeted to the Latino community. www.diabetes.org/DAR
- *African American Program:* diabetes awareness program targeted to the African American community. www.diabetes.org/africanamerican
- *Awakening the Spirit: Pathways to Diabetes Prevention & Control:* diabetes awareness program targeted to the Native American community. www.diabetes.org/awakening

To find out about an important research project regarding type 2 diabetes: www.diabetes.org/ada/research.asp

To obtain information on making a planned gift or charitable bequest: Call 1-888-700-7029. www.diabetes.org/ada/plan.asp

To make a donation or memorial contribution: Call 1-800-342-2383. www.diabetes.org/ada/cont.asp